STROKE AND STROKE RELATED DISORDERS IN THE ELDERLY

STROKE AND STROKE RELATED DISORDERS IN THE ELDERLY

NAGES NAGARATNAM AND
KUJAN NAGARATNAM

Rev. date: 04/09/2013

To order additional copies of this book, contact:
Xlibris Corporation
1-800-618-969
www.Xlibris.com.au
Orders@Xlibris.com.au
503126

CONTENTS

The Authors

Nages Nagaratnam, OAM, MD, FRACP, FRCPA, FRCP, FACC, FCCP is Clinical Associate Professor at the Sydney Medical School, The University of Sydney and Conjoint Associate Professor in the School of Medicine, College of Health and Science at the University of Western Sydney, Australia. He graduated and obtained the Doctorate in Medicine from the University of Ceylon and was for many years Consultant Physician in Internal Medicine in Sri Lanka and Senior Physician at the General Hospital, Colombo, the premier teaching hospital. He is a founding Fellow of the National Academy of Sciences of Sri Lanka and was President Section A of the Sri Lanka Association for the Advancement of Science. In Australia he was Consultant Physician in Geriatric and Internal Medicine at the Blacktown-Mount Druitt and Westmead Hospitals. He has an almost lifelong commitment to the training and guiding the careers of generation of young doctors. He has authored more than 200 scientific publications in both national and international journals. His interests spanned themes from many fields of medicine with continuous clinical research over several years. In the last two decades his interests are in geriatrics, rehabilitation, stroke and stroke rehabilitation.

Kujan Nagaratnam, MBBS (UNSW), FRACP graduated in Medicine from the University of New South Wales in 1988. He did his internal medical training and Advanced Training in Geriatric Medicine and Stroke Medicine at Westmead and Royal Prince Alfred Hospitals, Sydney. He obtained his Fellowship of the Royal Australasian College of Physicians (FRACP) in 1997. He held Senior Staff Specialist appointments in General, Geriatric Medicine and Stroke Medicine at Westmead Hospital and Blacktown—Mt Druitt Hospitaks until 2012. He is also Visiting Consultant Physician at The Norwest Private and Westmead Private Hospitals in Sydney. He is currently the Chairman and Head of the Department of Geriatric Medicine and Stroke Medicine, Norwest Private Hospital, Sydney. His academic interests includes teaching both undergraduate and postgraduate medical students. He is a Clinical Senior Lecturer in Medicine at The University of Sydney. His special interests are Stroke Medicine, Cognitive Impairment and Dementia, Neurological Diseases in the Elderly and Post-operative medical management of elderly patients.

Acknowledgements

We wish to thank Drs Senan Nagaratnam and Kevin Ng for the X'ray images. We would also like to thank Ms Angela Wallace, Sydney Medical School, Westmead, The University of Sydney and the Staff of the Blacktown-Mount Druitt Library for their help in labelling the line drawings. To Sai Nagaratnam and Manisha Nagaratnam for their help and above all to Isabel Nagaratnam a big thank you for her help with the Tables and putting everything together.

Disclaimer

Continuous development and research in the fields of medicine, science technology and health care result in on-going changes in the domains of clinical practice as evidence continues to evolve rapidly. We have taken reasonable care and effort to provide material which are current, accurate and balanced at the time of publication.

We and the publishers do not accept responsibility or liability for any errors in the text or any consequences arising from the information for instance to take the drug dosages as correct. The information provided is neutral and for general education and does not replace interaction with the practicing clinician. Clinicians should depend on their own experience when providing advice or treatment.

We have acknowledged the sources and works of the cited sites at the appropriate locations in the text and references. We have used the source materials in the sense of fair use and extend our apology for any oversight. Readers are advised to cross-reference and confirm points relevant to them.

1

INTRODUCTION

According to the World Health Organisation[1] most developed world countries have accepted the chronological age of 65 years, defined as 'elderly' or 'older person'. The elderly have been categorized as young old between the ages of 65 and 74 years, old old between 75 and 84 years and oldest old above 85 years and over[2]. The oldest old are the fastest growing segment of the population. The incidence of stroke increases with age and with increase in the life expectancy the older people will constitute a large portion of those afflicted with stroke. The proportion of stroke in the very old ranges from 4%[3] to 18.8%[4]. According to the Oxford Vascular Study there is a 12-fold increase in the incidence of acute ischaemic stroke in the age group >85 years compared to the younger population[5].

There is a progressive disability with age and those over the age of 80 years with stroke have a higher risk adjusted fatality, are associated with greater disability and functional impairment resulting in a high rate of institutionalization. The burden of stroke in the very old has been increasing in Western countries. There are age-based disparities in outcomes and measures to facilitate equal access for the elderly to specialized stroke care should be imposed[6]. It is tough to use age to judge general health and management options should not be determined solely on the basis of age[7]. An individual's behaviour should be regulated on the lifestyle which is influenced by personal and social characteristics, by cognitive capacity and the state of health and not merely on age.

Age-related changes should be distinguished from age-related or associated diseases. Diseases of old age are often considered distinct from changes associated with ageing. Ageing brings physiological changes that can affect the functional characteristics of individuals in this stage of life. In addition there are other factors concomitant with ageing that can influence negatively how elderly people function. Age-related changes in the heart vasculature, cerebral autoregulation are of significance to the development of stroke in the elderly[8]. Age-related changes, multiple co-morbidities and multiple medications can aggravate the insult from stroke and cause complications and prolong recovery.

Hippocrates (460-370 BC) was the first to recognize and describe stroke. The word *'apoplexia'* a Greek word meaning *'struck down by violence'* appeared in his writings and he described a patient with right arm weakness with loss of speech[9]. For several centuries little was known of the cause and treatment. The myth that someone suffering from stroke had been struck down by the gods, a divine retribution was widely believed. In the mid 1600s Johann Jakob Wepfer a Swiss physician first described carotid thrombosis and traced the carotid and vertebral arteries to the base of the brain. From his autopsy studies he noted that stroke is due to bleeding into the brain[9,10] and can also be caused by blockage of the arteries[11]. Stroke remained a neglected subject for several centuries for it was believed to be an unavoidable disorder with no credible treatment. There was a general feeling of despair and progression since then had been limited.

In more recent times stroke has attracted attention from the general public, the media and governmental agencies. This is associated with an increasing awareness of the significant burden of disability affecting the patient, his or her family and the enormous socio-economic burden that goes with it. It is only during the last 4 decades that there is an upsurge of interest in stroke-related clinical and research domains. This has largely been attributed to an emergence of a range of new knowledge in our understanding of stroke.

The primary event in the ischaemic cascade leading upto cerebral damage is the reduction of the cerebral blood flow. Unless there is adequate perfusion it would be difficult to achieve adequate concentrations of neuroprotective agent in the ischaemic area [12]. The 2-phase three National Institute of Neurological Disorders and Stroke (NINDS) tissue plasminogen activator trials completed in 1995 directly supported intravenous thrombolytic therapy in the the first 3-hours after stroke onset[13]. In a landmark re-analysis of the NINDS trials the pragmatic treatment effect in favour of tPA was established[14]. The safety and efficacy of intravenous thrombolysis in routine practice has been confirmed by the European Safe Implementation of Thrombolysis in Stroke Monitoring Study (SITS-MOST)[15]. Early intervention may be able to salvage moderate ischaemic areas (penumbra) that surround the more severe ischaemic area (core).

There is a paucity of randomized trials in the over 80 year group and most trials have excluded patients over the age of 80 years. The NINDS trial initialy restricted the age to 80 years but subsequently lifted the age criterion to include 42 patients over the age of 80 years[16,17]. The European Medicine Evaluation Agency did not approve thrombolytic therapy for patients over the age of 80 years for the reason that this group had been under-represented in major clinical trials[18]. Stroke patients in the age group of 80 years and over have a higher stroke mortality[19] without rtPA[20]and the mortality is twice as high in the over 85 years as compared to the under 85years [21]. Furthermore the outcome is worse[19]. The reasons for with holding thrombolytic therapy in the elderly ischaemic stroke patients are the dread of the risk of intracerebral haemorrhage, the poorer prognosis and greater in-hospital mortality[22, 23].

There are several studies with intravenous tPA in the very old patients with no increase in severe intracerebral haemorrhage [18,20,24] and the odds of beneficial outcome was as good as compared with the younger than 80 years of age group [25,26]. There are also studies that are at variance in that older patients recovery was less encouraging[19,27,28].

Data from the International Stroke Thrombolysis Registry (SITS-ISTR) and Virtual International Stroke Trials Archive (VISTA) when analysed revealed that those who underwent thrombolysis had significantly better functional outcome compared to those who did not and although increasing age was associated with poorer outcome, age alone should not be a barrier to treatment[29]. The Third Interntional Stroke Trial (IST-3) adds significant new input. The trial revealed that patients over 80 years attained similar benefit to those 80 years or younger with rt-PA, particularly when treated early[30]. The trial further showed that some younger patients might benefit within 6 hours of the stroke[30].

The advent of neuroimaging 4-5 decades ago has revolutionized neuroanatomy and neuroradiology. Our understanding of acute stroke pathophysiology has greatly improved with computerized tomography and magnetic resonance imaging—based perfusion imaging techniques. Diffusion-perfusion mismatch on MRI can provide a rough estimate of penumbral volume. They are now widely available. It helps with early diagnosis and provides precise information about the intravasculature, brain perfusion and facilitates the selection of appropriate therapy[31]. Neuroimaging has become an essential diagnostic criterion for stroke diagnosis. Advances in neuroimaging technology has resulted in an enormous degree of pathologic information in the clinical stroke setting.

One of the strategies that is gaining enormous acceptance is the creation specialized stroke care units. The initial concept of stroke intensive care units was first developed in the United States using the parallel model of acute intensive care units[32]. In a before-after analysis of cases treated in a standard community hospital care compared the results of patients in a neurovascular care unit found that the latter group had a 50% reduced complications[15]. The beneficial effect of stroke care units is now seen with the same measure of outcome across all age groups[33].

The most exciting area of development is in the field of stroke rehabilitation and the ever increasing evidence base has led to the expansion of methods and procedures to enhance better outcomes for stroke patients. Rehabilitation programmes emphasise functional retraining for the stroke survivors[34]. Currently the much spoken word in stroke rehabilitation is neuroplasticity. A wide range of potential interventions that may favourably modify outcome are being examined which include growth factors, electromagnetic stimulation, intense physiotherapy methods including constraint-induced movement therapy among others[35]. According to Hachinski[36] stroke in the next thirty years will be different in the fields of diagnostic precision and therapeutic importance.

CLINICAL RELEVANCE-Introduction

* There is a 12-fold increase in the incidence of acute ischaemic stroke in the age group >85 years compared to the younger population[5].
* It is tough to use age to judge general health and management options should not be determined solely on the basis of age[7].
* Age-related changes should be distinguished from age-related or associated diseases.
* Age-related changes for instance, in the heart vasculature, cerebral autoregulation are of significance to the development of stroke in the elderly[8].
* Stroke remained a neglected subject for several centuries for it was believed to be an unavoidable disorder with no credible treatment.
* In a landmark re-analysis of the NINDS trials the pragmatic treatment effect in favour of tPA was established[14].
* New data from the IST-3 trial confirmed rt-PA benefit to patients older than 80 years especially when treated early within the 3 hour window period with intravenous rt-PA[30].
* The reasons for with holding thrombolytic therapy in the elderly ischaemic stroke patients are the dread of the risk of intracerebral haemorrhage, the poorer prognosis and greater in-hospital mortality[22,23].
* Age alone should not be a barrier to treatment unless there are convincing evidence of unacceptable risk[29].
* Neuroimaging has become an essential diagnostic criterion for stroke diagnosis.
* The beneficial effect of stroke care units is now seen with the same measure of outcome across all age groups[32].
* Currently the much spoken word in stroke rehabilitation is neuroplasticity.

REFERENCES

1. World Health Organisation. Definition of older or elderly person. who/int/ healthinfo/survey/ageingdef-older/en/index/html.accessed on 25.01.2010.

2. Balducci L, Cohen HJ, Engstrom PF et al. Senior adult oncology, clinical practice guidelines in oncology. *J Natl Campr Canc Netw* 2005; 3: 72-75.

3. Agency for Health care Research and Quality: Health Care Utilization Project (HCUP) 1988-2000. *http://www.ahrq.gov/data/hc.up/hcup_pkt.htm*

4. Liebetrau M, Steen B, Skoog I. Stroke in 85 year olds: prevalence, incidence, risk factors and relation to mortality and dementia. *Stroke* 2003; 34: 2617-2620.

5. Rothwell PM, Coull AJ, Giles MF et al. Change in stroke incidence, mortality, case fatality, severity and risk factors in Oxfordshire UK from 1981-2004. (Oxford Vascular Study). *Lancet* 2004; 363: 1925-1933.

6. Bagg S, Pombo AO, Hopman W. Effect of age on functional outcomes after stroke rehabilitation. *Stroke* 2002;33;179-185.

7. Terret C. How and why to perform a geriatric assessment in clinical practice. *Ann Oncol* 2008; 19(Suppl 7): vii 300-3.

8. Shuaib A, Hachinski VC. Mechanism and management of stroke in the elderly. *CMAJ* 1991; 145(5): 433-443.

9. Thompson JE. The evolution of surgery for the treatment of stroke. The Willis Lecture. *Stroke* 1996; 27 (8):1427-34.

10. Storey CE, Pos H. Chapter 27: A history of cerebrovascular disease. *Handb. Clin Neurol* 2010;96:401-15.

11. Gurdijian ES, Gurdijian ES. History of occlusive cerebrovascular disease, I. from Wepfer to Moniz. *Arch Neurol* 1979;36(6):340-3.

12. Hussain MS, Shuaib A. Research into neuroprotection must continue . . . but with a different approach. *Stroke* 2008;39:521-522.

13. The National Institute of Neurological Disorders and Stroke rtPA Stroke Study Group: Tissue plasminogen activator for acute ischaemic stroke. *N Eng J Med* 1995; 333(24): 1511-7.

14. Ingall TJ, O'Fallon WM, Asplund K et al. Findings from the reanalysis of the NINDS tissue plasminogen activator for acute ischaemic stroke treatment trial. *Stroke* 2004; 39(10): 2418-24.

15. Quinn TJ, Lees KR. Advances in emerging therapies *Stroke* 2008; 39: 255-257.

16. Marlev R. Tissue plasminogen activator for acute ischaemic stroke. *NEJM* 1995;333:1581-1587.

17. Longstreth R, Katz DL, Tirschwell M. et al. Intravenous tissue plasminogen activator in stroke: an updated pooled analysis of ECASS, ATLANTIS, NINDS and EPITHET trials. *The Lancet* 2010;375:1695-1703.

18. Garcia-Caldentey J, de Lecinana MA, Simal P et al. Intravenous thrombolytic treatment in the oldest old. *Stroke Research Treatment* Vol 2012 (2012), Article ID 923676, 7 pages. Doi: 10.1155/2012/923676.

19. Berrouschot J, Rother J, Glahn J et al. Outcome and severe haemorrhagic complications of intravenous thrombolysis with tissur pladminogen activator in very old(>08 years) stroke patients. *Stroke* 2005;36:2421-2425.

20. Engelter ST, Bonati LH, Lyrer PA. Intravenous thrombolysis in stroke patients of >80 years versus <80 years of age-a systematic review across cohort studies. *Age Ageing* 2006;35(6): 572-580.

21. Kammersgaard LP, Jorgensen HS, Reith J, et al, Short and long-term prognosis for very old stroke patients. Ther Copenhagen Stroke Study. *Age Ageing* 2004;33:149-154.

22. Bateman BT, Schumacher HC, Boden-Albala B, et al. Factors associated with in-hospital mortality after administration of thrombolysis in acite ischaemic stroke patients: an analysis of the nationwide inpatient sample 1999 to *Stroke* 2006;37:440-6.

23. Heuschmann PU, Kolominsky-Rabas PL, Roether J et al. Predictors of in-hospital mortality in patients with acute ischaemic stroke treated with thrombolytic therapy. *JAMA* 2004;292:1831-8.

24. Ringleb PA, Schwark C, Kohrmann M et al. Thrombolytic therapy for acute ischaemic stroke in octogenarians: selection by magnetic resonance imaging improves safety but does not improve outcome. *J Neurol Neurosurg Psychiatry* 2007;78:690-3.

25. Engelter ST, Reichhart M, Sekoranja L et al. Thrombolysis in stroke patients aged 80 years and older. Swiss study of intravenous thrombolysis. *Neurology* 2005;65:1795-8.

26. Chen CI, Iguchi Y, Groth JC et al. Intravenous TPA for very old patients. *Eur Neurol* 2005;54: 140-4.

27. van Oostenbruge RJ, Huppetts RM, Lodder J. Thrombolysis for acute stroke with special emphasis on the very old: experience from a single Dutch centre. *J Neurol Neursurg Psychiatry* 2006;77: 375-7.

28. Sylaija PN, Cote R, Buchan AM, Hill MD. Thrombolysis for acute ischaemic stroke patients aged 80 years and older. Canadain Alteplase for Stroke Effective Study. *J Neurol Neurosurg Psychiatry* 2006;77

29. Mishra NK, Ahmed N, Andersen G et al. Thrombolysis in very old elderly people: controlled comparison of SITS International Stroke Thrombolysis Registry and Virtual International Stroke. *BMJ* 2010;341:c6046

30. Wardlow JM, Murray V, Berge E et al. The IST-3 collaborative group. Recombinant tissue plasminogen activator for acute ischaemic stroke: an updated systematic review and meta-analysis. *Lancet* 2-12; 379: 2364-72.

31. Srinivasan A, Goyal M, Al Azri F, Lum C. State of the art imaging of acute stroke. *Radiographics* 2006;26 (Suppl 1): S75-95.

32. JW, Hachinski VC. Intensive care management of stroke patients. *Stroke* 1976;7:595-7.

33. Saposnik G, Kapral MK, Coutts SB et al. Do all age groups benefit from organized inpatient stroke care? *Stroke* 2009; 40: 3321-3327.

34. Kollen B, Kwakkel G, Lindeman E. Functional recovery after stroke: A review of current developments in stroke rehabiliatation research. *Rev Recent Clin Trials* 2006; 1: 75-80.

35. Cramer SC, Riley JD. Neuroplasticity and brain repair after stroke. *Curr Opin Neurol* 2008; 21: 76-82.

36. Hachinski V. Stroke: The next 30 years. Editorial. *Stroke* 2002; 33: 1.

2

Overview of the anatomy
and functions of the brain

The brain is made up two cerebral hemispheres separated by the deep longitudinal fissure and connected by the corpus callosum. It is divided into three divisions, the forebrain, midbrain and hindbrain. In turn they are subdivided into four lobes, the frontal, parietal, occipital and temporal. In addition there is another, the insula which lies deep within the lateral central fissure. The lips of the lateral central fissure of the insula are called the opercula. The lateral central fissure (Sylvian fissure) separates the frontal lobe from the temporal and the central sulcus (fissure of Rolando) separates the parietal from the frontal. The parieto-occipital fissure separates the occipital lobe from the parietal lobe.

The basal ganglia lie deep within the cerebral hemispheres. It consists of the caudate which lies adjacent to the inferior border of the anterior horn of the lateral ventricle. Situated below the caudate and the insula is the lentiform nucleus which consists of the putamen lying just beneath the insular cortex and the globus pallidus lying medial to it. On either side of the third ventricle are the thalami. Lying below and ventral to them and forming the floor and part of the lateral wall of the third ventricle is the hypothalamus. The subthalmic nucleus is dorsolateral to the upper end of the substantia nigra and red nucleus. The substantia nigra and red nucleus extend into the caudal part of the mid-brain. Between the cerebral hemispheres and the pons is the mid-brain and ventral to the cerebellum is the pons. Between the pons and the spinal cord is the medulla oblongata.

Neural network

The neuron is the smallest structural element of the brain. There are three kinds of neurons, motor, sensory and interneuron. The neuron consists of a cell body with a highly arborized dendritic tree and axon. The dendrites receive information from other neurons or sensory receptors. The interneurons participate in feedback and forward back types of connections interrelating all of the cells linking both sides of the central nervous system. At the end of the axon is the axon terminal from where information which may be either excitatory or inhibitory is transmitted across the synaptic gap to the dendrites of the adjoining neuron. The information passes down from the cell body down the axon and travels in the form of an electrical signal known as action potential. The basic kinds of connections are chemical synapses and electrical gap. In some instances the electrical signal can bridge the gap (electrical gap). In other cases neurotransmitters are necessary[1].

The four primary neurotransmitters involved in maintaining a balanced brain are, acetylcholine, dopamine, gamma-aminobuytric acid (GABA) and serotonin. There is an age-related decline in the synthesis of the neurotransmitters and their receptors. At the cellular level neural death and neurochemical deficits occur in the cholinergic, serotonergic and GABA-nergic systems. Acetylcholine is widely distributed in the nervous system. The central cholinergic neurons project to a widespread areas of the cortex. The cholinergic neurons of the basal forebrain complex has been described to undergo moderate degenerative changes with aging[2]. Acetylcholine has been implicated to play a critical role in cortical activity, modulating cognitive performances, learning and memory processes[2].

About a hundred years ago Brodmann charted the structural and functional subdivisions in the brain which laid the basis for what is called the cytoarchitectonic organization of the brain cortex. The cortical map illustrates numerous areas in the brain as having specific and discrete functions. His numerical system attached to cytoarchitectonics were widely accepted[3]. Despite the fact that Brodmann's areas have been discussed, debated and refined over the years[4] a large number of investigators continue to use the Brodmann's map as a basis for the detection of physical and pathological processes.

Cerebral vascular anatomy

The cerebral hemispheres of the brain are supplied by the anterior, middle and posterior cerebral arteries. The arteries can be described in terms of segments. The internal carotid artery (ICA) terminates in the anterior (ACA) and the middle (MCA) cerebral arteries. Near the termination the ICA gives rise to the posterior communicating artery which joins caudally with the posterior cerebral artery. (PCA).

The carotids

The principal arteries that supply the brain are the common carotids, the vertebrals and the basilar arteries. The common carotids differ in length and their mode of origin. The innominate artery from the arch of the aorta gives rise to the right common carotid (CCA) and the right subclavian arteries. The left common carotid artery arises from the highest part of the aortic arch. The common carotid arteries ascend and divide into two branches namely the external carotid artery (ECA) and the internal carotid artery (ICA). The ECA supplies the exterior of the head, the face and greater part of the neck. Its main branches are the superficial temporal, internal maxillary and external maxillary arteries.

The ICA supplies to a large extent the cranial and orbital cavities. Internal carotid artery is described in segments namely cervical, petrous, lacerum, cavernous, clinoid, supraclinoid and communicating[5]. (Fig. 2.1). The opththalmic artery has two broad divisions namely the orbital and the ocular. The orbital group via the anterior and posterior ethmoidals and lacrimal branches supplies the orbital tissues. The lacrimal branch has important anastamosis with the middle meningeal artery. The ocular group through its branches the central retinal artery and long and short ciliary arteries supplies the ocular regions. The anterior choroidal artery arises from the ICA between the internal carotid bifurcation and the origin of the posterior communicating artery and its vascular territory shows variations but more commonly include the posterior limb of the internal capsule, optic tract, thalamus, lateral geniculate, medial temporal lobe and medial part of palllidum [6,7], uncus, amygdala, hippocampus and choroid plexus [8].

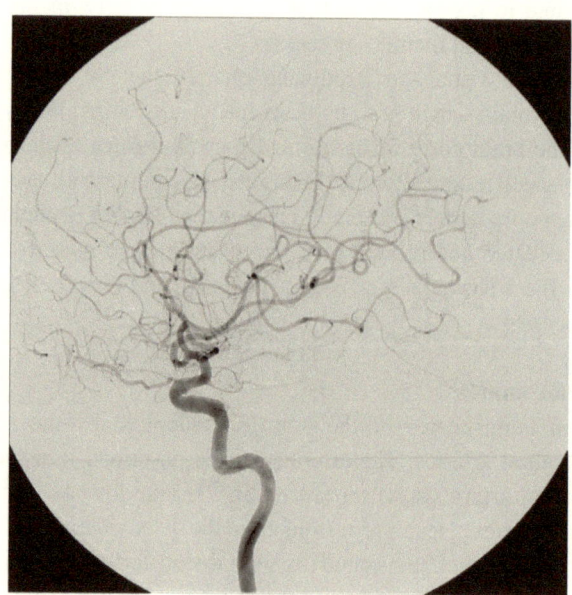

Fig 2.1. Cerebral angiography showing right internal
carotid artery and branches (anterior circulation)

Anterior cerebral artery (ACA)

The ACAs are connected via the anterior communicating artery. The first segment of the ACA is designated A1. The ACA supplies the medial surface of the cortex, frontal pole and anterior portion of the corpus callosum. The ACA gives rise to several prominent branches, the recurrent artery of Heubner, the orbito-frontal, the fronto-polar, arising near the anterior communicating artery complex[9], the callosomarginal and pericallosal, the last two supply the rostral sensorimotor cortex and the anterior 2/3rds of the corpus callosum (Fig 2.2 and 2.3). The medial lenticulostriate arteries arise from the A1 segment[10,11] and supply the anterior hypothalamus and adjacent structures. The recurrent artery of Huebner(RAH) normally arises from A1 segment [10,11] but may arise from A2 segment and most commonly from the junction of the ACA and the anterior communicating artery[12]. It supplies the anterior genu of the internal capsule, anterior third of putamen and the anteroinferior part of the head of caudate. A2 extends from the anterior communicating artery to the bifurcation forming the pericallosal and callosomarginal arteries. The orbitofrontal and fronto-polar arteries arise from this segment. The pericallosal artery termed A3 extends posteriorly to form the internal parietal and precuneus arteries. Callosomarginal bifurcates from the pericallosal and gives rise to or more major cortical branches[13] the medial frontal and paracentral arteries which supply the a portion of the parasaggital cortex of both lobes, medial aspect of frontal lobe and antero-medial aspect of the parietal lobe (Fig.2.2).

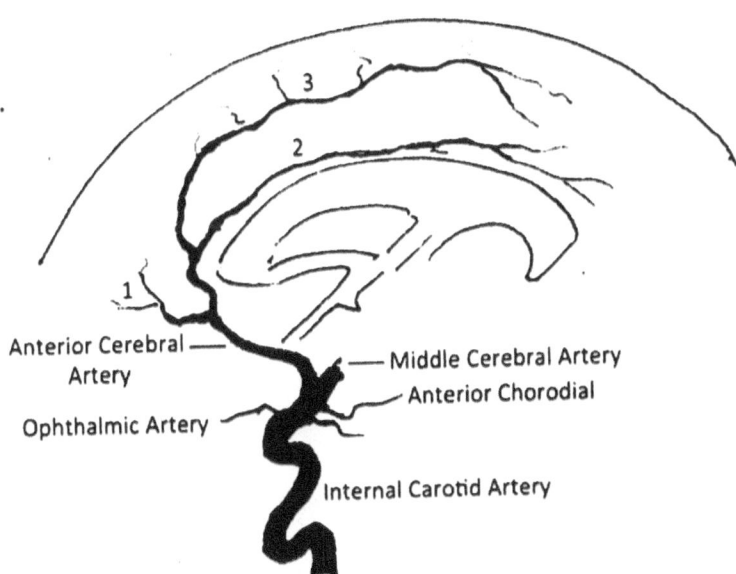

Fig.2.2. Diagram of the anterior cerebral artery and branches (medial view).
1. fronto-polar artery; 2. pericallosal artery; 3. calloso-marginal artery.

Middle cerebral artery (MCA)

The MCA enters the lateral cerebral fissure (Sylvian sulcus) and divides into cortical branches that supply the adjacent frontal, temporal, parietal and occipital lobes. Segmentally from the origin to the insula is M1. The horizontal portion of M1 gives rise to two and eight lenticulo-striate arteries which supply the head of caudate, putamen, lateral globus pallidus and the internal capsule except the posterior limb which is supplied by the anterior choroidal artery[8]. The anterior temporal branch also rises from M1 or may arise as part of the MCA trifurcation. M2 is the segment that runs along the insula and referred to as the 'insula segment'[14] of the MCA. M3, 'the opercular segment'[14] follows the insula to the operculum. The MCA bifurcates and enters the operculum as superior and inferior divisions. The superior division gives rise to 6 branches namely, lateral orbital, ascending frontal, precentral, central, anterior parietal and posterior parietal arteries. The inferior division gives rise to 3 branches namely, anterior, middle and posterior temporal arteries. M4, 'the cortical segment' [14] describes the branches of the MCA that perfuse the entire convex surfaces of the cerebral hemispheres. The cortical branches of the middle cerebral artery present fairly constantly are are the orbitofrontal, precentral, anterior parietal, precentral, posterior parietal, angular, posterior and anterior temporal arteries[14] (Figure 2.3 and 2.4).

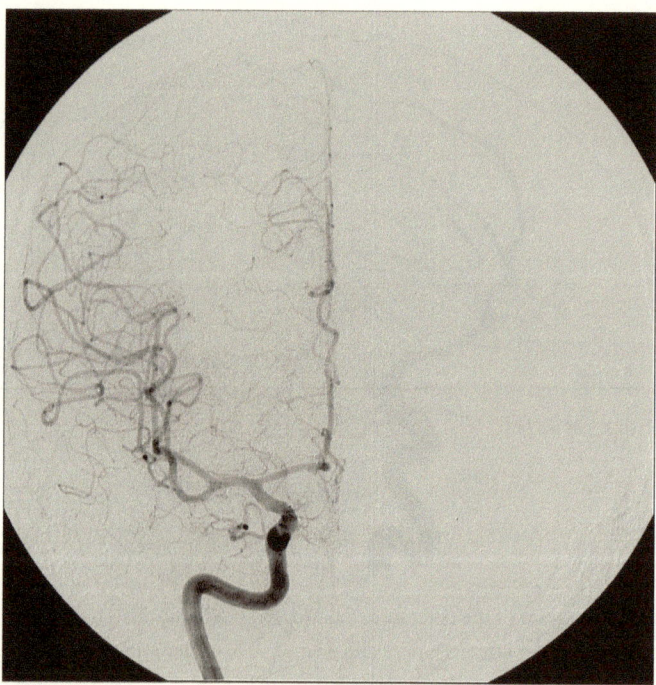

Fig 2.3. Cerebral angiography showing middle
and anterior cerebral arteries and branches

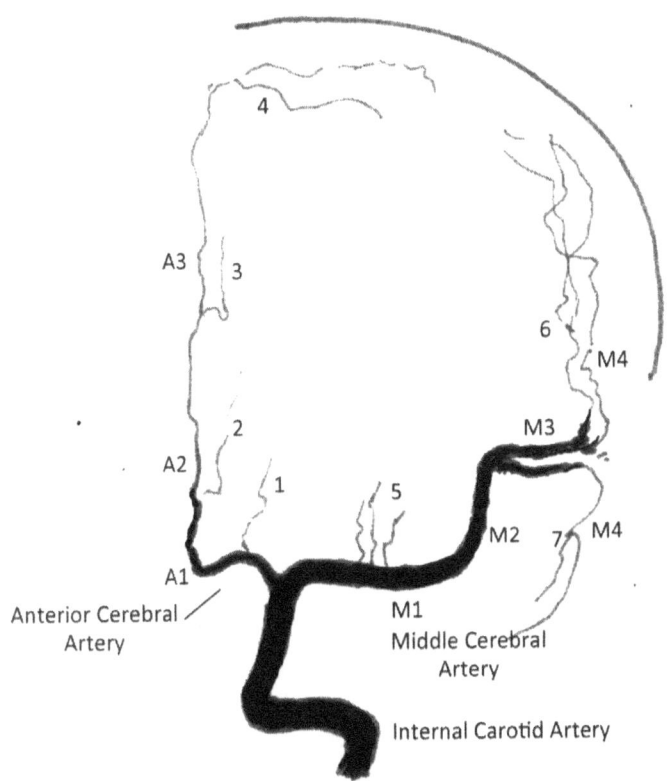

Fig.2.4. Diagram of the anterior cerebral and middle cerebral arteries and branches (posterior view).1. medial lenticulo-striate artery; 2. fronto-polar artery; 3. peri-callosal artery; 4. Callosomarginal artery; 5. lateral lenticulo-striate artery; 6. ascending fronto-parietal artery; 7. posterior temporal artery.

Posterior cerebral artery (PCA)

The right and left PCAs are formed from the bifurcation of the basilar artery near the front of the midbrain and pons. Each PCA can be divided anatomically into 4 segments (P1-P4). P1 extends from the origin of the PCA to the posterior communicating artery. P2 is the segment that courses around the mid-brain and its major branch, the lateral choroidal artery supplies the posterior thalamus. P3 and P4 are the distal branches which supply the cortical regions (Fig 2.5).

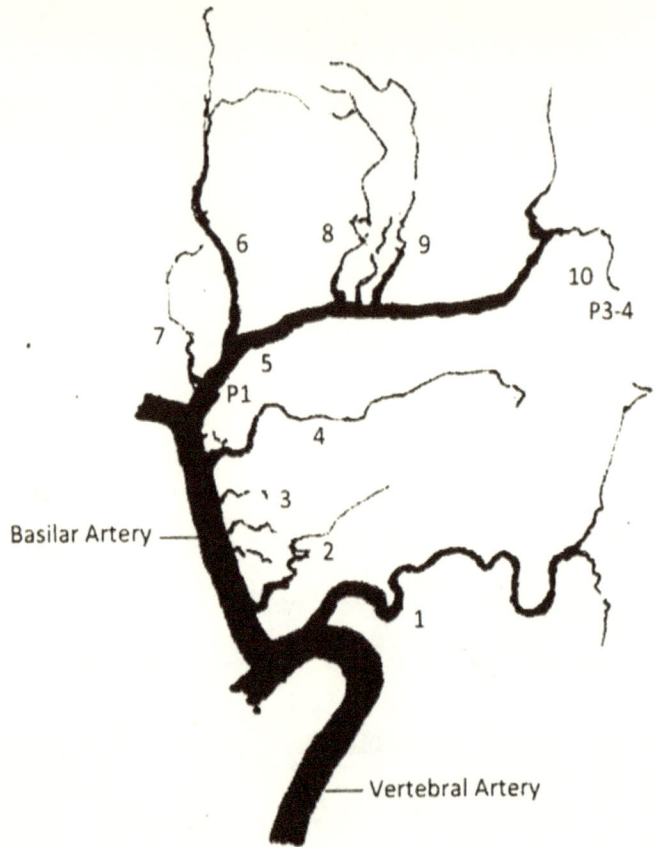

Fig 2.5. The vertebro-basilar system. 1. posterior inferior cerebellar artery; 2. anterior-inferior cerebellar artery; 3. pontine arteries; 4. superior cerebellar artery; 5. posterior cerebral artery; 6. posterior communicating artery; 7. paramedian artery; 8. medial posterior choroidal artery; 9. lateral posterior choroidal arteries.

Vertebro-basilar system

The right and left vertebral arteries are usually the first branches of the corresponding subclavian arteries. It gives rise to the posterior inferior cerebellar arteries (PICA) which runs around the medulla lying in the midline and thereafter runs posteriorly above the cerebellar tonsil to the under surface of the cerebellum. The basilar artery formed by the fusion of the two vertebral arteries and runs upwards in the midline of the pons terminating just above the tip of the dorsum sellae. It gives off branches on either side from below upwards the anterior inferior cerebellar arteries (AICA), superior cerebellar arteries, pontine arteries and the posterior cerebral arteries (PCA) (Fig.2.5 and 2.6).

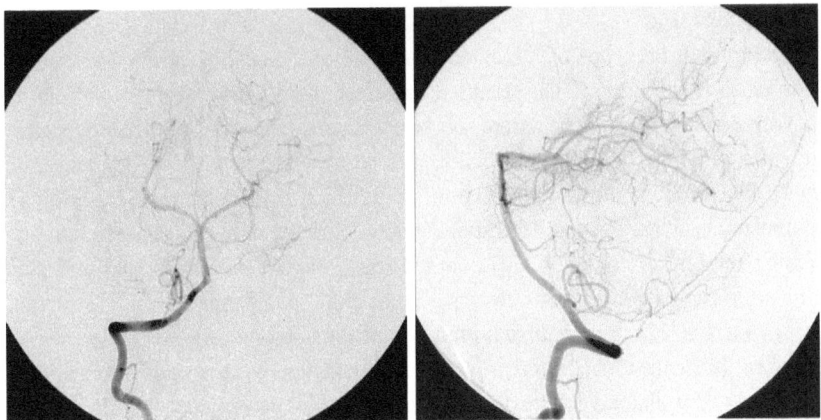

Fig 2.6. Cerebral angiography showing the
vertebrobasilar system (posterior circulation)

The AICAs run laterally on to the pons and anteroinferior surface of the cerebellum. Its branches include the internal auditory arteries and its cerebellar branches anastomose with the branches of the PCA. The right and left superior cerebellar arteries arise just below the PCAs. They run round the brain to fan out on the superior surface of the cerebellum. The basilar artery also gives about 12 pontine arteries that supply the medial pons. The basilar artery bifurcates to give rise to the PCAs. They run laterally and connecting with the posterior communicating arteries and then posteriorly surrounding the brain stem. Both PCAs and posterior communicating arteries give rise to the thalamaogeniculate and thalamo-perforating arteries. A medial posterior choroidal artery arise from the PCA to run around the midbrain and then curve over the pulvinar of the thalamus to reach the third ventricle. Two or more lateral posterior choroidal arteries arise along side and follow a similar course. The cortical branches of the PCA can be divided into two groups, the posterior temporal arteries and branches of the internal oocipital artery among which are the parieto-occiptal and inferior calcarine artery supplying the posterior third of the medial surface of the cerebrum including the visual cortex. They anastamose with the ACA anterosuperiorly and with the middle cerebral artery around the occipital pole.

Circle of Willis

Posteriorly the vertebrals arise from the subclavian arteries. The internal carotids and the vertebral arteries are directed at the base of the brain to form an anastomosis, the circle of Willis. The circle of Willis is formed in front by the anterior cerebral arteries, branches of the internal carotid arteries and connected together by the anterior communicationg artery and behind by the two posterior communicating arteries. Branches of the basilar arteries (posterior cerebral arteries) are connected on either side with the internal carotid arteries by the posterior communicating arteries. Several variations of the circle of Willis have been described[15].

Collateral pathways

The terminal branches of the anterior, middle and posterior cerebral arteries form the cortical arterial system. The terminal branches divide and ramify in the pia mater giving off branches which penetrate the brain cortex. The cranial collateral pathways include the (i) Circle of Willis, (ii) pial to pial pathways—the end—artery anastomosis on the surface of the brain from the anterior, middle and posterior cerebral arteries. These anastomosis occur via the so called meningeal or pial anastomosis between and among the major cerebral arteries and (iii) communication between the external and internal carotid arteries via ophthalmic artery reversed flow and from the middle meningeal branch of the ECA to the meningeal branches of the cerebral arteries[16,17]. In most cases of unilateral IC occlusion there is ipsilateral collateral flow via the ophthalmic artery and simultaneous contralateral collateral flow via the anterior communicating artery[16].

Border zones

About 10% of all cerebral infarcts are watershed infarcts[18]. Watershed areas occur in the distal fields of two non-anastamosing arterial systems that is the areas between the cortical supply of the ACA, MCA and PCA and referred to as the 'cortical watershed'[19] and the more rostral periventricular and supraventricular white matter of the corona radiata and the centrum semiovale referred to as 'internal watershed'[20]. The corona radiata is the watershed area between deep and superficial arterial systems of the MCA, and the centrum semiovale with the watershed zone between superficial system of the MCA and ACA. Infarction involving these areas are referred to as 'terminal supply infarcts' or 'inner or subcortical watershed infarcts[20].

Neuroplasticity

Stroke results in damage in the brain. Brain recovery may take place by several mechanisms. Neuroplasticity refers to the brain's ability to restructure itself by collateral sprouting from intact cells to dennervated region or unmasking of neural pathways and synapse formation not only in the spared regions of the damaged hemisphere but also in the hemisphere contralateral to the injury[21,22]. The brain can reorganize existing pathways by taking over the function in some other area or the adjacent spared tissue are altered in a functionally modified network.

During the execution of motor tasks the elderly manifest greater brain activation than younger controls [23]. The investigators hypothesized that this age—related 'overactivation' could be to compensate for the various neural and behavioural deficits in the aging brain[23]. Alternately they felt it could be a 'dedifferentiation' due to deficits in neurotransmission reflecting a nonfunctional spread of activity[23]. Aging is associated with deficits in a number of functional domains including cognition, memory, motor control and sensation [24]. Studies of adult brain plasticity using properly designed behavioral training practices has shown improvement in these areas [24].

* The cerebral hemispheres of the brain are supplied by the anterior, middle and posterior cerebral arteries.
* The cranial collateral pathways include the Circle of Willis, the communication between the external and internal carotid arteries and the pial to pial pathways—the end—artery anastomosis on the surface of the brain from the anterior, middle and posterior cerebral arteries which penetrate the the brain cortex.
* The neuron is the smallest structural unit and the interneurons participate in feedback and forward back types of connections interrelating all the cells linking both sides of the central nervous system
* Neurons communicate with each other by means of synapses and the basic kinds of connections are chemical synapses and electrical gap.
* The neurotransmitters are generally categorized into four groups, acetylcholine, monoamines (dopamine, serotonin, epinephrine and norepinephrine), amino acids (glycine, gamma-aminobutyric acid—GABA, glutamate) and peptides.
* Brodmann's areas have been discussed, debated and refined over the years and Brodmann's map continue to be used for the localization of physical and pathological processes.
* The brain's ability to restructure itself after injury is referred to as neuroplasticity. Aging is associated with continuing functional deficits in areas of cognition, motor control, sensation, memory among others[24].
* Studies in adult neuroplasticity have shown that appropriately contrived behavioural practices could improve function and or recovery in these areas[24].

REFERENCES

1. Cherry K. About.com.Guide. What is a Neuron?. *http://psychology/.about.com/od/biopsychology/f/neuron.01.htm* retreived 12.10.12
2. Schliebs R, Arendt T. The cholinergic system in aging and neuronal degeneration. *Behav Brain Res* 2011;221:555-563.
3. Pearce JMS. Broadmann's cortical maps. *J Neurol Neurosurg Psychiatry* 2005;76:259.
4. Broadmann Area. Ed Frederic P. Miller, Agnes T Vandone, John McBuster, Alphascript Publishing.2010
5. Bouthillier A, van Loveren HR, Keller JT. Segments of the internal carotid artery: A New Classification. *Neurosurg* 1996;38(3):425-432.
6. Carpenter MB, Noback CR, Moss ML. The anterior choroidal artery—It's orogin course and distribution and variations. *Arch Neurol Psychiatry* 1954;71:714-22.
7. Hegalson C, Caplan LR, Goodwin H, Hedges III T. Anterior choroidal artery-territory infarction: report of cases and review. *Arch Neurol* 1986;43:681-6.
8. Vu D. Blood supply of the CNS (Lecture notes) University of New South Wales 26 October 1998, http://download.videohelon/vitualis/med/blood_supply.brain.htm
9. Avci E, Fosett D, Aslan M et al. Branches of the anterior cerebral artery near anterior communicating artery complex: an anatomic study and surgical perspective. Neurol Med Chir (Tokyo) 2003;43:329-3 (abstract).
10. Rhoton AL. The supratentorial arteries. *Neurosurg* 2003;51(Suppl 1):53-120
11. Krayenbuhl HA, Yasargil MG. Cerebral angiography. 2nd ed. English ed New York, Thieme Medical Publishers,1968;20-85
12. Loukas M, Louis RG, Jr, Childs RS. Anatomical examination of the recurrent artery of Huebner. *Clin Anat* 2006;19(1):25-31 (abstract).
13. Cavalcanti DD, Albuquerque FC, Silva DF et al. The anatomy of the callosomarginal artery: applications to microsurgery endovascular surgery. Neurosurg 2010;66(3):602-10 (abstract).
14. Pai SB. Varma RG, Kulkarni RN. Microsurgical anatomy of the middle cerebral artery. *Neurology India* 2005;53:186-190.
15. Kapoor, K, Singh B, Dewan IJ. Variations in the configuration of the circle of Willis *Anat Sci Int* 2008;83:96-106 (abstract).
16. Love L, Hill BJ, Larson SJ et al. Cranial collateral pathways in stroke syndrome. *Am J Roentgenology* 1966; 98: 637-646.
17. Liebeskind DS. Collateral circulation. *Stroke* 2003;34:2279-2284.
18. Torvik A. The pathogenesis of water shed infarcts in the brain. *Stroke* 1964;15(2):221-223.
19. Mangala R, Koler B, Almast J, Ekholm SE. Border zone infarcts: Pathophysiology and imaging characteristics. *Radiographics* 2011;31:1201-1214.

20. Momjian-Meyer I, Barod J-C. The pathophysiology of watershed infarction in internal carotid artery disease. *Stroke* 2005:31:567-577.

21. Bagg S, Pombo AO, Hopman W. Effect of age on functional outcomes after stroke rehabilitation. *Stroke* 2002;33:179-185.

22. Kozlowski DA, Schaller T. Relationship between dendritic pruning and behavior recovery following sensorimotor cortex lesions. *Behav Brain Res* 1998;97:89-98

23. Heuninckx A, Wenderoth N, Swinnen SP. Systems Neuroplasticity in the aging brain: recruiting additional neural resources for successful motor performance in elderly persons. *J Neurosci* 2008;28(7):91-99.

24. Mahncke HW, Bronstone A, Merzenich MM. Brain plasticity and functional losses in the aged: scientific bases for a novel intervention. *Prog Brain Res* 2006;157: 81-109.

3

EPIDEMIOLOGY OF STROKE
IN THE ELDERLY

Stroke has become an enormous public health problem in almost every nation and is the leading cause of mortality and morbidity worldwide. According to the World Health Organisation stroke is the most common severe neurological disorder and the third leading cause of mortality in adults[1]. It is a leading cause of morbidity and mortality in Western countries[2]. Demographic and epidemiological trends suggest the stroke in the elderly will be a major health issue in the near future with significant cost implications.

Incidence

The incidence of stroke rises exponentially with increasing age. About half of all strokes occur in the group aged >70 years and nearly a quarter occur in those who are >85 years of age[3,4]. The incidence rates of first-ever stroke rose markedly with age and will keep increasing even at 90 years and over[5]. The incidence of all strokes doubles with each decade after the age of 55 years. The Rotterdam Study showed an incidence rate of stroke per 1000 person years increased with age and ranged from 1.7 in men aged 55 to 59 years to 69.8 in men aged 95 years or over. In women it was 1.2 and 33.1 respectively[6].

The overall age and sex standardized incidence rates to the 1991 European population were 8.72 per 1000 person years aged 65 to 84 yers and 17.3 per 1000 person years for those 75 years and over[5]. The overall prevalence of stroke age and sex adjusted in the same study was 4.84% in the 65-84 years individuals and 7.07 in those 75 years and older[5]. While people age 85 years and over had relatively lower incidence of cardiovascular risk factors they suffered stroke with a very high frequency and had a higher death rate[7].

Geographical

Several studies have suggested geographical disparities. Comparisons of stroke incidence within countries and communities and between countries is useful to identify high risk populations. The incidence rate of stroke in an Australian population study from Melbourne was similar to that of European studies but was significantly higher than that observed in the West coast of Australia[8]. A prospective community based stroke register including all age groups in Germany revealed the incidence rates were similar to that reported for population-based studies in Western industrialized countries[9]. It was however lower in the former East Germany[9]. Comparable studies in Norway revealed incidence rates of stroke were similar to that of other Scandinavian countries and comparison between other European countries did not indicate any regional variations with Western Europe[10]. The European Registers of Stroke (EROS) Investigators found the risk of stroke from data obtained from population—based stroke registers among European populations on average had higher rates of stroke in the eastern and lower rates in southern European countries[11]. Another community-based stroke incidence study of a Scottish population(Scottish Border Stroke Study) found the crude incidence rate as one of the highest in the world but adjusted rates, case fatality and relative risk for all strokes and stroke subtypes were not significantly different from the majority of other stroke studies[12].

In the United States there are regional differences, the stroke incidence was highest in the south eastern states ('Stroke Belt') compared to the south western and highly populated north eastern states[13]. Analysis of self—reported data from the 2005 to 2007 comparing 153106 respondents from the Stroke Belt region with 6615 cases of stroke vs 612262 respondents with 21347 cases from non—Stroke Belt region found the stroke prevalence was 1.25[14]. It is felt that known risk factors and socioeconomic status accounted for the difference in stroke prevalence[15]. Compared to New Zealanders and Europeans, the Maori/Pacific Islanders, Asian and other migrants are at higher risk of ischemic stroke and primary intarcerebral haemorrhage whereas similar rates of subrachnoid haemorrhage were evident in all ethnic gropus[16].

Race

Caucasians have higher rate of coronary artery disease (CHD) and lower prevalence of stroke as compared with Asians[17]. The prevalence rates of stroke in Western countries in the 1980s were 500-700 per 100,000[18] and in Asians 900 per 1000,000[19]. Population based surveys in stroke from different parts of India showed the aged-adjusted annual incidence rate during the last decade to be 105/100,000 in the urban community of Kolkata and the demographic and epidemiological trends suggest the stroke in the elderly will be a major health issue in the near future with significant cost implications [20]. The age adjusted annual incidence rate was 105/100,000 in the urban community of Kolkata[20] and 262/100,000 in the rural community in West Bengal [21]. The age—adjusted incidence of first-ever stroke in mainland China from community surveys of six cities in 1983 was 219/100,000 population higher in the north than in the south[17]. The age adjusted annual incidence rate in the West is between 100 to 300 per 100,000 populations [22].

Mortality and morbidity

Stroke is the third leading cause of death in the United States[23]. It is the leading cause of mortality and morbidity in the elderly. 90% of all stroke cases are in people who are 55 years or older and the death rate doubling every ten years between 55 and 85[23]. Age—adjusted death rate for whites males have declined from approximately 100/100,000 in 1979 to 50/100.000 in 1998. While stroke mortality rates have declined the numer of total strokes deaths have increased in the US in the 1990s. This is because the rate of decline slowed and the number of elderly in US has increased dramatically. This trend may continue as the percentage of older people continues to increase[23]. In the United Kingdom too the stroke mortality rates have been falling from the late 60s but as a consequence of its ageing population the burden of stroke may increase[24].

Stroke mortality varies considerably by race and sex and there are geographic differences. In general males have a slightly higher age adjusted stroke rate than females[23]. Blacks have a very high stroke mortality rate. While stroke mortality is declining in US, worldwide it is increasing along with modernization and stroke rates in Eastern Europe have been increasing.

The rule of the thumb is one-third of the stroke patients die. Of the remaining two-thirds half are significantly disabled and the remaining half capable of independent living. In the United States annual estimate is 731,000 strokes and 4 million survivors[25]. The burden of stroke is not distributed equitably around the United Kingdom, the mortality rates were higher in the North of Engand, Wales and Scotland compared to South of England and whether this due to incidence or case fatality is unclear[26].

Stroke type

The Australian—the North East Melbourne Stroke Incidence Study (NEMESIS) found 72.6% with cerebral infarction, 14.5% with intracerebral haemorrhage, 4.3% subarachnoid haemorrhage and 8.7% of the undetermined type in 381 strokes. The case fatality in thae same study was 12% for cerebral infarction, 45% for intracerebral haemorrhage, 50% for subarachnoid haemorrhage and 38% for stroke of the undetermined type[27]. A two-year community—based study from Joinville, Brazil of 759 first ever strokes, 610 (80.3%) had infarction, 94 (12.4%) intracerebral haemorrhage and 55 (7.2%) subarachnoid haemorrhage[28]. In a recent study of 474 intracerebral haemorrhage patients the men had poor outcome within 28 days. In the 75 years of age and younger 20% women and 23% of men died compared to 26% and 41% in the 75 years and older respectively[29].

Stroke of uncertain cause is the most common subtype of ischaemic stroke among American blacks and cardioembolic and small vessel stroke were the most common identifiable causes among blacks[30]. A population-based study from Southern Italy recorded a lower incidence of cerebral infarction to other population-based studies from Northern European and United States [31]. Lacunar infarction was the most common ischaemic stroke subtype in Japan (54%)[32] and in Pakistan (42.7%)[33]. In the Japanese population the age-adjusted incidence rates for lacunar 77.1, cardio-embolic 31.5 and non-lacunar $29.7/10^5$ [32]. Second to lacunar infarction, large vessel atherosclerosis accounted for 36.9%, followed by undetermined 20.3% and cardio-embolic 6.1% in Pakistan[33].

Risk factors

Cardiac arrhythmias are a large concern among the elderly and they occur so frequently that they are often regarded as 'normal' and inevitable part of normal ageing[34]. More recently the large Atherosclerosis Risk in Communities (ARIC) study showed the occurrence of premature ventricular complexes were associated with new-onset atrial fibrillation and death[35]. Atrial fibrillation (AF) is a relatively common arrhythmia. Risk factors for AF include age, male gender, hypertension, valvular disease and coronary artery disease among others and the last three are the most common predisposing conditions in the elderly. Among the heart diseases that increase the incidence of AF are the valvular disease especially mitral stenosis, mitral incompetence and tricuspid incompetence. The Framingham Heart Study examined 5184 men and women to determine the impact of AF on the risk of stroke with increasing age in a 30 year follow up[36] showed that AF was a significant contributor to stroke at all ages. Chronic AF (without valvular disease) appeared in 303 individuals. The age-specific incidence rates increased from 0.2 per 1000 for ages 30 to 30 to 39.0 per 1000 persons ages 80-89 years. The proportion of strokes associated with AF was 14.7% [36]. The stroke rate increased steadily with age from 6.7% from ages 50-59 years to 36.2% ages 80-89 years[36].

Other specific risk factors for stroke include, the left ventricular mass (as determined by echocardiography)—to-height was found to have a hazard ratio for cerebrovascular events of 1.4 for each quartile increment after adjustment for age and sex[37]. Carotid medial wall thickness is a surrogate measure of subclinical atherosclerosis and is a strong predictor of future stroke[38]. Increased carotid artery intima thickness[39,40] and plaque characteristics[40] were found to be risk factors for stroke in the elderly. The Northern Manhattan study reported a greater stroke risk with prevalent irregular carotid plaques, an approximate 5 times increased risk of stroke[41].

The cardiovascular health study [41] found that both internal carotid artery intima thickness and elevated C-Reactive Protein(CRP) were associated with the occurrence of ischaemic stroke. In another community-based, multi-ethnic, stroke-free cohort study in North Manhattan high sensitivity CRP (hsCRP) measurements in 2240 individuals age 40 years and older were examined. Those with hsCRP levels more than 3mg/L were at increased risk for ischemic stroke compared to those with levels less than 1mg/L after adjustment for risk factors[42].

There has been several reports[43,44,45] of the link between socio-economic differences and stroke risk in the elderly. The Rotterdam study revealed a strong association among elderly women between socio-economic status and stroke and the association was only partly explained by known risk factors[46]. It was emphasized that strategies for primary prevention of stroke should target less affluent people[45]. Avendano et al[44] found lower socioeconomic status was associated with higher stroke incidence for both income and education at ages 65 to 74 years. Beyond the age of 75 the stroke rates were higher among those with highest education and income which remained largely unchanged after adjustment for risk factors.

Besides environmental factors for stroke there is a genetic component. Family history of stroke is known to be an independent risk factor for stroke and studies involving twins, siblings and families have detected evidence of hereditability but to date the identification of genes involved is unclear [40]. Genetic markers may be of interest in helping to understand the factors that influence the predisposition to stroke. High von Willibrand Factor (v WF) levels increased the risk of first ischaemic stroke[47] and is associated with increased risk of stroke in the general population[48]. vWF is synthesized by the endothelial cells and plays an important role in platelet adhesion to the subendothelial structures and is a useful marker of endothelial dysfunction[49].

* The incidence of stroke increases exponentially with increasing age and increasing even at 90 years and over[5]
* Age, race and sex are all strong risk factors.
* There are geographical variations in the incidence and mortality world-wide with ethnic and regional differences.
* Family members have a genetic tendency for stroke.
* Modifiable risk factors include heart disease (myocardial infarction especially invoving the anterior wall, left ventricular hypertrophy, atrial fibrillation, carotid artery disease, hypertension, diabetes mellitus area are at high risk of stroke.
* There has been several reports on socio-economic differences and stroke in the elderly[43-45].
* About 90% of all stroke cases are in people who are 55 years and older and the death rate doubles every ten years between 55 and 85 years.
* Cardiac arrhythmias are a large concern among the elderly and the occurrence of premature ventricular complexes have been shown to be associated with new-onset AF and death[34].
* Increased carotid artery intima thickness and plaque characteristics were found to be risk factors for stroke in the elderly[39,40].

REFERENCES

1. WHO Stroke 1989: Recommendations on stroke prevention, diagnosis and therapy. Report of the WHO task force on stroke and other cerebrovascular disorders. *Stroke* 1989; 20: 1407-1431.
2. Sarti C, Rastenyte D, Cepaitis Z, Tuomilento J. International trends in mortality from stroke. 1968-*Stroke* 2000; 31: 1588-1601.
3. Bramford J, Sandercock P, Dennis M et al. A prospective study of acute cerebrovascular disease in the community, the Oxfordshire Community Stroke Project 1981-86-1: methodology, demography and incidence increase of first ever stroke. *J Neurol Neurosurg Psychiatry* 1988; 51: 1373-1380.
4. Brown RD, Whisnsant JP, Sicks D et al. Stroke incidence, prevalence and survival: recent trends in Rochester Minnesota through *Stroke* 1996; 27: 373-380.
5. Di Carlo A, Launer LJ, Breteler MMB et al. Frequency of stroke in Europe: A collaborative study of population based cohorts. ILSA working Group and the Neurological Diseases in the Elderly Research Group: Italian Longitudinal Study on Ageing. *Neurology* 2000; 54(11 Suppl5): S34-7.
6. Hollander M, Kondstaal PJ, Bots ML et al. Incidence, risk and case fatality of first ever stroke in the elderly population. The Rotterdam Study. *J Neurol Neurosurg Psychiatry* 2003; 74: 317-321.
7. Pozsegovitis K, Kazu OS, Nagy Z. et al. Epidemiology of stroke in the elderly. *Ideggyogy Sz* 2006 NW20, 59(11-12): 449-53.
8. Thrift AG, Dewey HM, Macdonell RH et al. Stroke incidence on the East coast of Australia: the North East Melbourne Stroke Incidence Study (NEMESIS). *Stroke 2000*; 31(9): 2187-92.
9. Kolomensky-Rabas PL, Sarti C, Henschmann PU et al. A prospective community-based study of stroke in Germany-the Erlangen Stroke Project (ESPrO): incidence and case fatality at 1.3, and 12 months. *Stroke* 1998; 29(12): 2501-6.
10. Ellekjaer H, Holmen J, Indredavik B, Terent A. Epidemiology of stroke in Innherred, Norway 1994-Incidence and 30-day case fatality rate. *Stroke* 1997; 28: 2180-2184.
11. The European Registers of Stroke (EROS) Investigators. Incidence of stroke in Europe at the beginning of the 21st century. *Stroke* 2009; 40: 1557-1563.
12. Syme PD, Byrne AW, Chen R et al. Community-based stroke incidence in a Scottish population: the Scottish Border Stroke study. *Stroke* 2005; 36: 1837-43.
13. Rich DQ, Gaziano JM, Kurth T. Geographical patterns in overall and specific cardiovascular disease in apparent healthy men in the United States. *Stroke* 2007; 38: 3221-3222.
14. Liao Y, Greenland KJ, Croft JB. et al. Factors explaining excess stroke prevalence in the US Stroke Belt. *Stroke* 2009; 40: 3336-3341.
15. Truelson T. Advances in population-based studies. *Stroke* 2010; 41: e99-e101.

16. Feigin VL, Carter KN, Anderson C et al. Ethnic disparities in incidence of stroke subtypes, the Auckland regional community stroke study 2002-*The Lancet Neurology* 2006; 5: 130-139

17. Li SC, Schoenberg BS, Wang C et al. Cerebrovascular disease in the People's Republic of China: epidemiologic and clinical features. *Neurology* 1985; 35: 1708-13.

18. Kurtzke JF. Epidemiology of cerebrovascular disease. In Sickert RG. ed Cerebrovascular Survey. Report of the Joint Council of the Subcommittee on cerebrovascular disease. National Institute of Neurological and Communicable Disorders and Stroke and the National Heart and Lung Institute, Rochester, Minnesota: Whiting Press, 1980: 135-76.

19. Wallin MT, Kurtzke JF. Neuroepidemiology. In: Bradley WG, Daroff RB, Feinichel GM et al rds: Neurology in Clinical Practice. Philadelphia: Butterworth Heinemann, 2004: 763-79.

20. Banerjee TK, Mukherjee CS, Sarkhel A. Stroke in the urban population of Calcutta-an epidemiological study. *Neuroepidemiology* 2001; 20: 201-7.

21. Bhattacharaya S, Saha SP, Basu A, Das SK. A 5-year prospective study of incidence, morbidity and mortality profile of stroke in a rural community of Eastern India. *J Indian Med Assoc* 2005; 103: 655-9.

22. Banerjee TK, Kumar S K. Epidemiology of stroke in India. *Neurology Asia* 2006;11:1-4.

23. American Heart Association, 2001 Heart and Stroke Statistical Update, Dallas, Texas: *Amer Heart Assoc*, 2000.

24. National Audit Office. *Health Focus Spring*. National Audit Office,2009.

25. Broderick J, Brott T, Kothari R et al. The Greater Cincinnati/Northern Kentucky Stroke Study. *Stroke* 1998; 29:415-421.

26. Bhatnagar P, Scarborough P, Smeeton NC, Allender S. The incidence of all stroke and stroke sub-type in the United Kingdom 1985-A systematic review. *BMC Public Health* 2010;10:539.

27. Thrift AG, Dewey HM, Macdonell RAL et al. Incidence of major strole types. Initial findings from the North East Melbourne Stroke Incidence Study (NEMESIS). *Stroke* 2001; 32: 1732-1738.

28. Cabral NL, Goncalves ARR, Longo AL. et al. Incidence of stroke subtypes, prognosis and prevalence of risk factors in Joinville, Brazil: a 2-year community based study. *J Neurol Neurosurg Psychiatry* 2009; 80: 755-761.

29. Zia E, Eugstrom G, Svensson PJ et al. Three year survival and stroke recurrence rates in patients with primary intracerebral haemorrhage. *Stroke* 2009; 40(11): 3567-73.

30. Woo D, Geisal J, MillerR et al. Incidence rates of first ever ischaemic stroke subtypes among blacks-a population based study. *Stroke* 1999; 30: 2517-2522.

31. Manobiaco G, Zoccolella S, Petruzellis A. et al. The incidence of major stroke subtype in Southern Italy: a population based study. *Eur J Neurol* 2010;17:1148-1155.

32. Turin TC, Kita Y, Rumana N et al. Incidence stroke subtypes in a Japanese population-Takashima Stroke Registry 1988-*Stroke* 2010;41:187-96

33. Syed NA, Khealani BA, Ali et al. Ischaemic stroke subtypes in Pakistan. The Aga Kahn University Stroke Data Bank. *JAMA* 2003; 53: 584-6.

34. Fulberg CD, Psaty BM, Manolio TA et al. Prevalence of atrial fibrillation in elderly subjects (the Cardiovasdcular Health Study). *Am J Cardiol* 1994; 74: 236-241.

35. Agarwal SK, Heiss G, Rautaharju PM et al. Premature ventricular complexes and risk of incident stroke: the Atherosclerosis Risk in Communities (ARIC) Study. *Stroke* 2010; 41: 588-593.

36. Wolf PA, Abbott RD, Kanal B. Atrial fibrillation: A major contribution to stroke in the elderly. *Arch Intern Med* 1987;147(9): 1561-1566.

37. Bikkina M, Levy M, Evans JC et al. Left ventricular mass and risk of stroke in the elderly cohort. The Framingham Heart Study. *JAMA* 1994; 272(1): 33-36.

38. Humphries SE, Morgan L. Genetic risk factors for stroke and carotid atherosclerosis: insights into pathophysiology for candidate gene approaches. *The Lancet Neurology* 2004; 3(4): 227-238.

39. Cao JJ, Thach C, Manolio TA et al. C-Reactive Protein Carotid Intima Media Thickness and incidence of ischaemic stroke in the elderly. The Cardiovascular Health Study. *Circulation* 2003; 108: 166-170.

40. Kitamura A, Iso H, Imano H et al. Carotid Intima-Media Thickness and Plaque characteristics as a risk factor for stroke in Japanese eldely men. *Stroke* 2004; 35: 2788-2794.

41. Prabhakaran S, Rundek T, Ramas R et al. Carotid plaque surface irregularity predicts ischaemic stroke: The Northern Manhattan Study. *Stroke* 2006; 37: 2696-2701.

42. Elkind MS, Luna JM, Moon YP. et al. High-sensitivity C-reactive protein mortality but not stroke.: the Northern Manhattan Study. *Neurology* 2009; 73: 1300-1307.

43. Hart CL, Hole DJ, Smith GD. The contribution of risk factors to stroke differentials by socioeconomic poor in adulthood. The Renfren/Parsley Study. *Am J Public Health* 2000; 90(11): 1788-1791.

44. Avendano M, Kawachi I, Van Lenthe F et al. Socioeconomic status and stroke incidence in the US elderly. *Stroke* 2006; 37: 1368-1373.

45. Cesaroni G, Agabiti N, Forastiere F, Perucci CA. Socioeconomic differences and stroke incidence and prognosis under a universal health care system. *Stroke* 2009; 40(8): 2812-9.

46. Van Ramussen CTM, van deMheen H, Breteker MB et al. Socioeconomic difference in stroke among Dutch elderly women. The Rotterdam Study. *Stroke* 1999; 30: 357-362.

47. Bongers T, de Maat M, van Goor M et al. High von Willebrand Factor levels increase the risk of first ischaemic stroke. Influence of ADAMTS13. inflammation and genetic variability *Stroke* 2006; 37(11): 2672-7.

48. Wieberdink RG, van Schie MC, Kondstaal PJ et al. High von Willibrand Factor levels increase the risk of stroke. The Rotterdam study. *Stroke* 2010; 41: 2151-2156.

49. Sato M, Suzuki A, Nagata K, Uchiyama S. Increased von Willibrand Factor in acute stroke patients with atrial fibrillation. *J Stroke Cerebrovasc Dis* 2006; 5(1): 1-7.

4

PATHOPHYSIOLOGY AND PATHOGENESIS

Approximately 15% of strokes are due to primary intracerebral hemorrhage one-third of which is subacrachnoid haemorrhage and the remaining 80-85% to cerebral infarction. About 25% of the ischaemic strokes are due to atherosclerosis and may follow hypoperfusion or atherogenic embolism. Small vessel disease giving rise to lacunar infarcts amounts to 25%[1]. A further 25% (ranging from 14-30%)[2] are due to cardiac embolism and the remaining to a number of causes namely, arteritis, dissection among others (Fig 4.1 and 4.2).

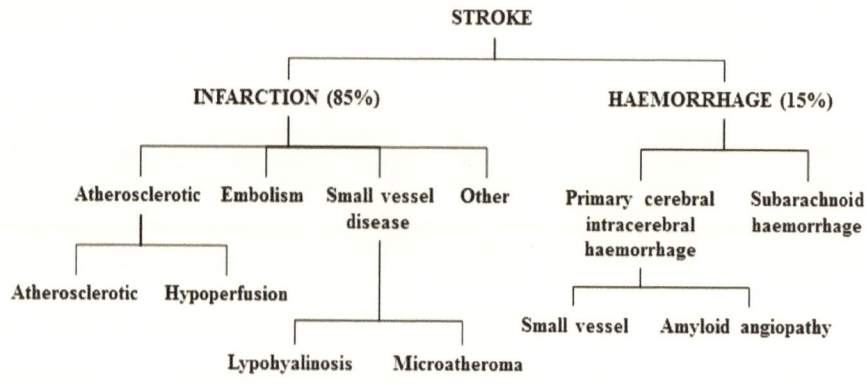

Fig.4.1 Causes of stroke

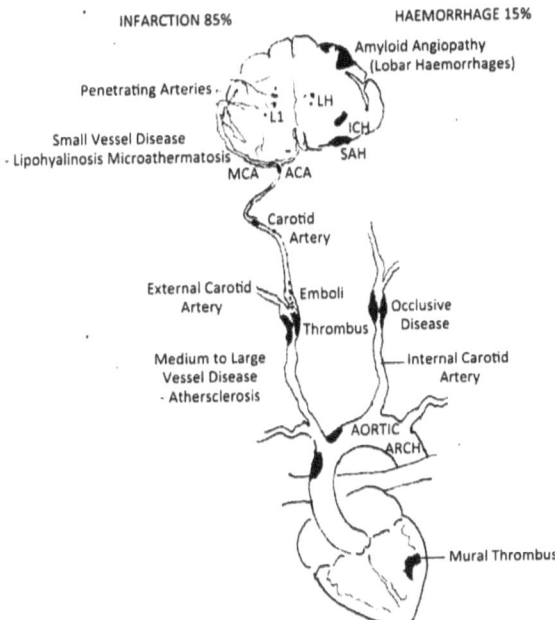

Fig.4.2. Pathophysiology of stroke

CEREBRAL INFARCTION

Large vessel atherosclerosis

Atherosclerosis is by far the commonest pathological feature resulting in stroke. Atherosclerosis is primarily typified by the formation of intimal plaques called *atheroma*. A chain of events leads upto the formation of the plaque. The early steps however remains largely disputed. Several theories have been proposed to explain the initial and subsequent growth of the atheromatous plaque. Many of the events are linked to at least initially to chronic injury to the endothelium[3]. According to the insudation theory the focal accumulation of fat in the vessel wall is derived from the plasma lipoproteins. This begins with endothelial dysfunction which may be triggered by factors such as shear stress and turbulent flow, oxidative stress, hyperlipidaemia, hypertension, smoking, impaired glucose metabolism among others[3,4]. The endothelium has two important roles, one is that it prevents the passage of substances in the blood into the vessel wall and the other it prevents intravascular clotting.

Oxidative stress is said to have an important role in the causation of endothelial dysfunction[5,6]. Increased production of oxidative radicles not only cause dysfunction of the endothelial cells but also oxidation of low density lipoprotein and migration of monocytes and smooth muscle cell growth. Sheer stress have been shown experimentally to increase endothelial permeability[7]. Insudation of the lipoproteins mainly the Low Density Lipoprotein (LDL) into the intima undergo modification and initiates monocyte migration to localize in the intima and promote differentiation of monocytes into macrophages. The lipoproteins are taken up by the monocytes to become lipid filled foam cells the hall mark of atherosclerosis[8,9]. Further plaque progression involves more macrophages and formation of a core of extracellular lipid and cholesterol within the plaque. The endothelial cells, macrophages and smooth muscle cells (SMC) release chemotactic growth factors which stimulate proliferation of SMC of intimal or medial origin. These cell components produce excessive connective tissue matrix[10] and results in the formation of a mature fibrous plaque. The accumulation of SMC and extracellular matrix and formation of the central core of extracellular lipid characterises the complicated atheromatous plaque[9]. Overlying the lipid core is the fibrous cap. Neovascularization is another contribution to plaque growth. These vessels can rupture as they are fragile giving rise to haemorrhage within the plaque and sudden expansion of the plaque[11,12].

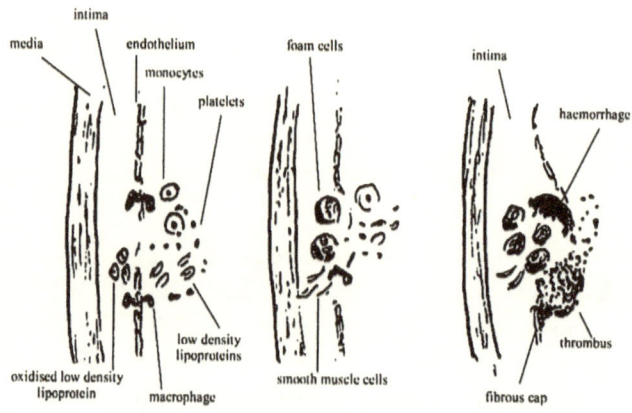

Fig.4.3 Atherosclerosis and Thrombus formation

As the plaque evolves denudation of the endothelium occurs followed by platelet deposition giving rise to the release of platelet derived growth factor (PDGF) which further enhances the proliferation of SMC [13]. The loss of endothelium allows thrombi to form over the plaque(superficial), With plaque rupture the thrombus forms within the plaque (deep). The fibrous cap of the plaque tears to expose the lipid core containing large amounts of cholesterol crystals, fragments of collagen and tissue factor and thrombus forms rapidly within the plaque itself[14].

The plaques (i) may undergo patchy or massive calcification, (ii) may fissure or ulcerate and may develop superimposed thrombus, (iii) may rupture and discharge debris into the blood stream, and (iv) the loss of endothelial integrity may invoke haemorrhage either an influx of blood from the vessel lumen or arise from peripheral capillaries. The haemorrhage could balloon the plaque and cause its rupture. Damage to the underlying media may result in atherosclerotic aneurysm[15].

Thrombus formation

The thrombogenic cascade is triggered as the result of endothelial injury. The formation of the arterial thrombus involves platelet adhesion and platelet aggregation. Activation and accumulation of the platelets are triggered by injury (erosion/ denudation) to the endothelium exposing the collagen allowing platelets to adhere to it. Platelet activation also occurs with the release of Tissue Factor derived from the atherosclerotic plaque. Arterial thrombus is said to occur in two discrete stages[16]. Adhesion and aggregation of platelets on the collagenous plaque components which include fibronectin, von Willibrand Factor (vWF) and collagen are mediated by GP-Ia/IIb and Glycoprotein (GP) VI[11]. Under high shear-stress conditions von Willibrand Factor (vWF) appears to play an important role in both platelet adhesion and aggregation[17].

At the same time the coagulation cascade is initiated by the formation of thrombin and fibrin which is triggered by the Tissue Factor which is independent of vWF and glycoprotein[18,19]. The release of Tissue Factor activates Factor X which in turn activates the generation of thrombin from prothrombin. Thrombin converts fibrinogen to fibrin Thrombin plays a vital role in activating platelets and also causes platelets to changes shape and stick to each other [20]. Enhanced exposure and activity is the final common pathway of clot formation[14]. Continuing platelet to platelet adhesion using the IIb/IIIa receptor and fibrinogen as binder the platelet areas grow. The early platelet mass is unstable but with the conversion of fibrinogen to fibrin it becomes secure[20].

Activated platelets release two substances which contribute to increased expression of IIb/IIIa receptor. One is thromboxane A2 (TXA2) which can be blocked by aspirin and the other is adenosine diphosphate (ADP) which also stimulates platelet recruitment. Clopidergrol acts by inhibiting the binding of ADP to its platelet receptors and more specifically to the low affinity receptors, the high binding receptors remain unaffected[21].

Cellular mechanisms of neuronal death

Occlusion emboli, atherosclerotic or other vascular diseases of the cerebral artery leads to focal cerebral infarction. Ischaemia is rapidly followed by neuronal cell death. Neuronal function is damaged in two stages. Firstly, cerebral blood flow (CBF) normally about 50ml blood/100gm/minute falls to about 20ml blood/100mg/minute and normal function is endangered but is reversible. An area called the penumbra may result, a region which is potentially salvageable[22] by early re-perfusion. If the CBF falls below 10 ml blood/100gm/minute and the brain tissue membranes remained unrelieved by restoration of normal blood flow or by the development of collateral circulation they will lose their ability to maintain electrolyte or other gradients between intracellular and extracellular fluid and irreversible damage occurs with death of the neuronal cells, a central core of infarcted tissue results [22].

There has been a new understanding of the mechanisms by which ischaemic neurons die. In cerebral ischaemia there are three cellular mechanisms for cell death—necrosis, apotosis and neuroptosis. Arterial occlusion results in reduction of blood flow depriving the brain of oxygen (hypoxia) and glucose (hypoglycaemia) and this leads to the development of an ischaemic injury. This follows a breakdown of cellular integrity through a series of intricate cellular events brought about by ionic imbalance, oxidative stress and cellular dysfunction [23,24].

Limiting the cerebral blood flow leads to oxygen deprivation causing a decrease in the levels of adenosine triphosphate (ATP)[25,26] and results in an inability to maintain electrochemical gradients. ATP is essential for the functioning of Na+/K+ ATPase and changes in the concentration gradient of Na+ and K+ results in a release of glutamate[27] and excess glutamate results in excitotoxicity[24]. Excitotoxicity can lead to apoptotic or necrotic cell death. There is an increase in the levels of glutamate after stroke[28] and a persistence release leads to progression of the infarction. The activation of the excitatory amino acids is mediated by opening of the receptor gated ion channel, the N-methyl-D-aspartate (NMDA). This results in rapid increase in intraneuronal cytosolic Ca $2+$[29] ceasing protein systhesis. The increase in the intraneuronal calcium concentration is detrimental to the neuronal cell causing it to swell, rupture with leakage of the contents into the surrounding tissue and cell death[30,31]. With prolonged or complete ischaemia, neuronal death is inevitable and is now known that secondary biochemical changes that occur in response to the intial result worsen the injury.

Ischaemic injury can also be exacerbated by the inducible proteins that mediate programmed cell death (PCD). PCD pathways are reported to be present in the penumbra[32]. Neurons are 'programmed' to die under certain conditions such as ischaemia. The ischaemia activates latent 'suicide' proteins in the nuclei which triggers an autolytic process resulting in cell death. This autolytic process is mediated by DNA cleavage[33,34]. Before death the neurons undergo characteristic changes associated with apoptosis[35].

There are other cell death pathways activated during stroke[32]. Stroke injury leads to a cell death program through activation of poly(ADP-ribose) polymerase-1 (PARPI) and ending in an apoptosis inducing factor (AIF) mediated cell death[36]. Other factors studied in AIF release in stroke are calcium-dependent protease (calpain) and cycophalin A[32].

Fig 4.4 is a schematic diagram illustrating the main molecular mechanisms leading up to neuronal death following ischaemic injury. Although generally cell death is classified into two forms, apoptosis also known as PCD and necrosis [37,38] it is incorrect to infer that apoptosis and PCD are the same because cell death can manifest non-apoptotic features during physiological development[39]. Necroptosis is a mechanism which embraces both necrotic and apoptotic components.

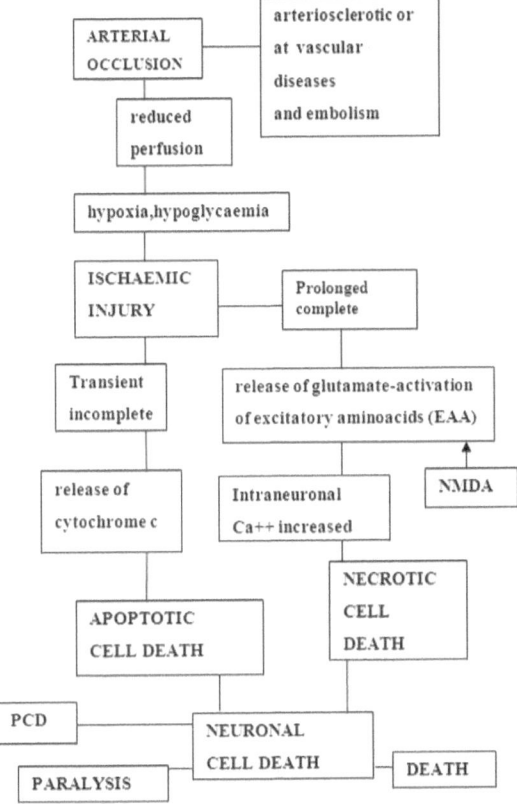

Fig.4.4 Modified schematic illustration of neuronal cell death at the molecular level in infarction. PCD: Programmed Cell Death; NMDA: N-methyl-D-aspartate

Information sources: Choi et al [29], *Graham and Hickey [30], Kajsutra et al [33] (*with permission from ACNP)

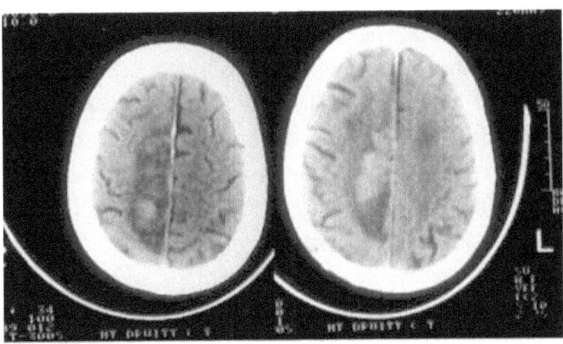

Fig.4.4. Haemorrhagic infarction in the territory
of the right anterior cerebral artery

II. Small vessel disease

It is widely surmised that disease of the small intracranial vessels are responsible for the small deep seated (lacunar) infarctions and primary cerebral haemorrhages[40]. About 25% of ischaemic strokes are due to small vessel disease following occlusion of the small penetrating arteries. Fisher[41] distinguished two types of underlying vascular pathology, lipohyalinosis and microatheromatosis. The vessels that are affected by lipohyalinosis measure 40-210 μm in diameter. The lacunar infarcts vary in size measuring 3-20μm and are found in the caudate, putamen, thalamus, internal capsule, pons and white matter of the cerebellum[41]. They are usually asymptomatic. The penetrating vessels are usually end arteries and the area supplied by the vessels have limited collateral flow. Lipohyalinosis is characterized by loss of normal arterial architecture, formation of mural foam cells and in acute lesions evidence of fibrinoid wall necrosis[42]. Lipohyalinosis should not be confused with concentric wall thickening, a feature of aged brains especially those with hypertension and diabetes[40]

The other vascular lesion involves somewhat larger perforating arteries (200-800 μm) and commonly cause larger infarcts[41]. They are more often symptomatic and particularly involve the striatocapsular region. According to Fisher[43] the atheromatous plaques are seen in the proximal portion of the perforating artery at its origin or in the parent artery. Infarctions are related to occlusive plaques rather than to compression by overlying thrombosis. Leukoaraiosis or periventricular white matter hypodense on CT scan are also caused by lipohyalinosis of the white matter perforating small arteries[42]. Leukoaraiosis is associated with hypertension[44].

PATHOGENESIS

I. Ischaemic stroke

In cerebral infarction, the mechanisms are i. Embolism-the embolic material originating from the heart (cardio-embolic) or from non-cardiac source, for instance, the carotid arteries (artery to artery embolus). ii. Thombotic-formation of a thrombus or clot within a cerebral vessel. iii. Thromboembolic-embolic material originating from a thrombus. iv. Haemodynamic: hypoperfusion giving rise to border zone/ watershed infarction. Within an hour of the ischaemic insult there is an area of severe ischaemia known as the 'core zone'. There is necrosis of the neurons as well as the supporting glial cells. Surrounding this area is an ischaemic zone of oligaemia called the 'penumbra'. The extent of the penumbra varies with the rate and duration of the ischaemic event and number and patency of the collaterals. Other factors which may influence the progression of the ischaemic injury are inadequate systemic blood pressure, elevated body temperature, low or high blood sugar.

Changes that may occur following cellular injury during the ischaemia is brain oedema. There are two types of oedema, cytotoxic and vasogenic[45]. Cytotoxic oedema occurs within minutes to hours and the main feature is the swelling of the cellular elements of the brain parenchyma and swelling of the astrocytes the main form[46].

Cytotoxic oedema may not necessarily be permanent. Hypoxia resulting from acute cerebral ischaemia causes the cellular elements to swell due to failure of the ATP dependant (Na and Ca) transport. The rapid accumulation of sodium within the cells results in flow of water to maintain osmotic equilibrium increasing the cell volume.

In contrast the vasogenic oedema results from disruption of the blood brain barrier[45,47]. The vasogenic oedema occurs over hours to days and is considered to be irreversible. It is characterized by increase in the extracellular fluid volume due to increased permeability of the capillary endothelial cells resulting in influx of plasma proteins and fluid collecting in the extracellular spaces[47]. It can give rise to mid-line shift and to cerebral herniation. Larger the infarct the greater the potential to develop cerebral oedema.

Cerebral oedema also initiates oxidative and inflammatory cascades resulting in disruption of the blood brain barrier, vasogenic oedema and haemorrhagic transformation[48]. An ischaemic infarct can undergo haemorrhagic conversion or transformation. Haemorrhagic transformation occurs in approximately one-third of cases of ischaemic stroke[49]. Haemorrhagic conversion can take two forms, haemorrhagic infarction(HI) and parenchymatous haematoma (PH). HI is confined within the vascular territory, is usually asymptomatic and on CT scan appears as hyperdense areas ranging from a few petechiae and patchy to confluent areas of bleeding[50] (Fig.4.5). PH differs from HI in that it extends beyond the vascular territory, is symptomatic, often exerts mass effect and on CT appears as hyperdense homogenous collection of blood[50]. In most instances PH is due to rupture of an ischaemic vessel which has been subject to reperfusion pressures[50]. The differentiation between haemorrhagic infarction and primary intracerebral haemorrhage can be difficult especially if the imaging is delayed after the onset of the patient's symptoms[51].

CEREBRAL HAEMORRHAGE

Pathophysiology

Approximatey 80% of primary intracerebral haemorrhage (PICH) is due spontaneous rupture of small vessels damaged by hypertension. Second most common cause is cerebral amyloid angiopathy. Seconday intracerebral haemorrhages are due to either congenital causes or acquired conditions such as vascular anomalies, coagulopathies, various drugs among others.

Cellular mechanisms of neuronal death

Cerebral haemorrhage is a dynamic process and continues for several hours. Many of the haemorrhages continue to expand over several hours after the onset of symptoms. In a third of the patients it occurs within the first 24 hours and in two-thirds of them it is evident within the first 4 hours[52]. The expansion is likely to be due to continued bleeding from the primary source and to mechanical disruption of the surrounding vessels. A local coagulation deficit and acute hypertension may be associated[53]. Inflammation caused by thrombin and end products of coagulation causes most of the brain injury and swelling[54]. Haematoma initiates neuronal damage and oedema which accumulates in the extravascular space[55] results from the osmotically active proteins in the haematoma, develops over the first 24-96 hours and slowly resolves over several weeks. The late—onset oedema which persists for several weeks after the initial haemorrhage is the result of disruption of the blood brain barrier. Neuronal death occurs in the regions surrounding the haematoma and is predominatly necrotic and there is evidence to suggest the presence of programmed cell death (apoptosis)[54] (Fig.4.6).

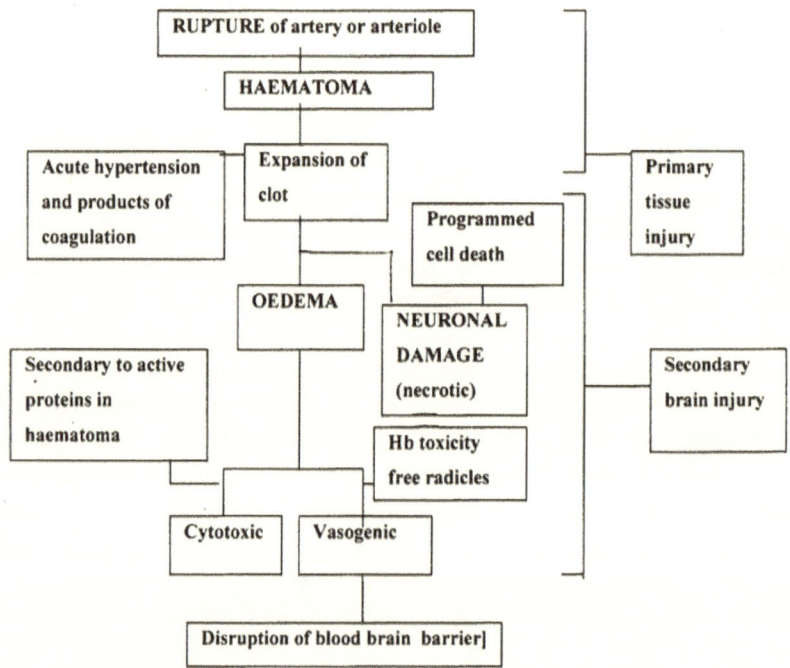

Fig 4.6 Modified schematic illustration of neuronal death at molecular level in cerebral haemorrhage

Information sources: Brott et al[52]; Qureshi et al[53];* Chakravathy and Shivane[54] *Major source with permission from ACNR, Butcher et al[55].

I. Small vessel disease

In microvascular disease the small penetrating arterioles of the subependymal and pial microvasculature tend to become stenosed or they may dilate to form microaneurysms. Hypertension causes fibrinoid necrosis[56] and hypertension increases the formation of microaneurysms[57]. It is the fibrinoid changes in the arterioles that lead to the formation of microaneurysms and rupture. Patients with microvascular brain disease can have recurrent events which can be either ischaemic or haemorrhagic. The formation of microanuerysms make the haemorrhagic events more frequent. They are found more frequently in the putamen, globus pallidus, thalamus and less frequently in the internal capsule, caudate nucleus and subcortical white matter[58]. It is surmised that sudden alterations in cerebral blood flow or pressure cause fibrinoid necrosis and cause vessel to rupture[40].

II. Cerebral amyloid angiopathy (CAA)

CAA results from extracellular deposition of fibrillar proteins (b-amyloid or Ab) on the walls (tunica media and adventitia) of small and mid-sized blood vessels of the brain and leptomeninges[59]. The deposition of Ab occurs in the cortical and leptomeningeal vessels[60] resulting in fibrinoid necrosis and formation of microaneurysms. Age is the strongest risk factor for CAA and is a major cause of ICH and the haemorrhages occurred at microaneurysms with fibrinoid necrosis[61]. The haemorrhages are superficial, lobar cerebral[61,62] and cerebellar [63] and often breach the cortical surface resulting in secondary subarachnoid haemorrhage[61]. They can be multiple and recurrent. The most frequent sites of CAA related haemorrhages are the occipital and frontal lobes[64] with subcortical haemorrhages. MRI may show petechial cortical and subcortical haemorrhages even in patients who are asymptomatic[65]. Other features are leucoencephalopathy[66] and small cortical ischaemic infarcts. CAA is common in the elderly and is often found in association with Alzheimer's disease[67]. 83% of 117 brains of patients who had confirmed Alzheimer's disease had evidence of CAA[68].

Diagnosis during life is impeded by the need for post-mortem examination for definite diagnosis. Using a combination of clinical, radiological and pathological data, the Boston Criteria was developed which aided and reliably differentiated lobar intracerebral haemorrhage into categories of possible, probable or definite based on the likelihood of underlying CAA[69] (Fig.4.7).

CLINICAL RELEVANCE—
PATHOPHYSIOLOGY AND PATHOGENESIS

* Atherosclerosis is by far the commonest pathological feature resulting in stroke and is typified by the formation of intimal plaque called atheroma.

* About 25% of ischaemic strokes are due to small vessel disease following occlusion of the small penetrating arteries, the pathology being lipohyalinosis or microatheromatosis.

* Cerebral ischaemia may result in a central core of infarcted tissue surrounded by a region which is potentially salvageable called the penumbra.

* In cerebral ischaemia there are three cellular mechanisms for cell death namely, necrosis, apoptosis and neuroptosis.

* Understanding of the mechanisms of neuronal death in relation to ischaemia continues to evolve.

* About 80% of primary intracerebral haemorrhage is due to spontaneous rupture of small vessels damaged by hypertension.

* CAA is common in the elderly and is often found in association with Alzheimer's disease [67].

* The Boston criteria reliably differentiates lobar intracerebral haemorrhages into categories of possible, probable and definite based on the likelihood of underlying CAA[69].

REFERENCES

1. Sudlow CLM, Warlow CP. Comparable studies on the incidence of stroke and its pathological types. Results from an international collaboration. *Stroke* 1997;28:491-9.
2. Arboix A, Alio J. Cardioembolic stroke: clinical features, specific cardiac disorders and prognosis. *Curr Cardiol Rev* 2010;6(3): 150-161 (abstract).
3. Boyle EM Jr, Lille ST, AllaireE et al. Endothelial cell injury in cardiovascular surgery: atherosclerosis. Ann Thorac Surg 1009;63(3):885-94 (abstract).
4. Reiner Z, Tedeschi-Reiner E. New information on pathophysiology of atherosclerosis. Lijec Vjesn.2001;123(1-2):266-31 (abstract)
5. Wadsworth R. Oxidative stress and the endothelium. *Exp Physiol* 2008;93:155-157 (abstract).
6. Hugashi Y, Noma K, Yoshimi M, Kihara Y. Endothelial function and oxidative stress in cardiovascular diseases. *Circ J* 2009;73(3):411-8 (abstract).
7. Ogunrinade O, Kameya GT, Truskey GA. Effect of fluid sheer stress on permeability of the arterial endothelium. *Ann Biomed Eng* 2002;30(4): 430-46 (abstract).
8. Tegos TJ, Kalodiki E, Sabetai MM et al. The genesis of atherosclerosis and risk factors: A review. *Angiology* 2001; 52: 89-94.
9. Libby P, Geng YJ, Aikawa M et al. Macrophages and atherosclerotic plaque stability. *Curr Opin Lipidol* 1996;7(5): 330-5(abstract).
10. Mitchell ME, Sidawy AN. The pathophysiology of atherosclerosis. *Semin Vasc Surg.* 1998;11(3):134-41 (abstract).
11. Virmani R, Kolodgie FD, Burke AP et al. Atherosclerotic plaque progression and vulnerability to rupture: angiogenesis as a source of intraplaque haemorrhage. Atheroscler *Thromb Vasc Biol* 2005;25(10):205-211 (abstract).
12. Di Stefano R, Felice F, Balbarini A. Angiogenesis as a risk factor for plaque vulnerability. *Curr Pharm Des* 2009; 15(10):1095-106 (abstract).
13. Rainer EW. PDGF and cardiovascular disease. *Cytokine & Growth Factor Reviews* 2004;15:237-254 (abstract).
14. Davies MJ. Arterial thrombosis and acute coronary syndromes in Acute Coronary Syndromes. *Amer Coll Cardiol* June 1999.
15. Kumar V, Contran RS, Robbins SL. Basic Pathology. Fifth Ed. WB Saunders Co. Philadelphia. 1992.
16. Reininger AJ et al. A two step mechanism to arterial thrombus formation induced by human atherosclerotic plaques. *J Am Coll Cardiol* 2010;55:1147-1158
17. Jansson HH, Nilsson TK, Johnson O. von Willibrand factor in plasma: a novel risk factor for recurrent myocardial infarction and death. *Br Heart J* 1991;66:351-5.

18. Dubois C, Panicot-Dubois L, Merrill-Skoloff G. et al. Glycoprotein VI-dependent and—independent pathways of thrombus formation in vivo. *Blood* 2006;107:3002-

19. Dubois C, Panicot-Dubois L, Gainor JF et al. Thrombus initiated platelet activation in vivo is von Willibrand factor independent during thrombus formation in a laser injury model. *J Clin Invest* 2003;117:453-60.

20. Brass LF. Thrombin and platelet activation. *CHEST* 2003, 124:185-255.

21. Savi P, Nurden P, Nurden AT et al. Clopidergrol: a review of its mechanism of action. *Platelets* 1998;9(3-4):251-255.

22. Liang D, Bhatta S, Gerranich V, Simard JM. Cytotoxic oedema: mechanisms of pathological swelling. *Neurosurg Focus* 2007 May 15.22(5)EE.

23. Lo EH, Dalkara T, Moskovitz MA. Mechanisms challenges and opportunities on stroke. *Nat Rev Neurosci* 2003;4:2003.

24. RR, Baron J-C. Pathophysiology and therapy of experimental stroke. *Cell Mol Neurobiol* 2006;20:1057-1083.

25. Kastura K, Kristian T, Siesjo BK. Energy, metabolism, ion homeostasis and cell damage in the brain. *Biochem Soc Trans* 1994;22:991-996.

26. Martin RL, Lloyd HG, Cowan AI. The early events of oxygen and glycose depletion: setting the scene of neuronl death? *Trends Neurosci* 1994;17: 251-257.

27. Rothman SM, Olney JN. Glutamate and pathology of hypoxic-ischaemic brain damage. *Ann Neurol* 1980;19:105-111.

28. Bullock R, Zanner A, Woodward J, Young HF. Massive persistent release of excitatory aminoacids following human occlusive stroke. *Stroke* 1995;26:2187-2189.

29. Choi DW, Koh JY, Peters S. Pharmacology of glutamate neurotoxicity in cortical cell culture: attenuation by NMDA antagonists. *J Neurosci* 1988; 8: 185-196.

30. Graham SM, Hickey RW. Molecular pathophysiology of stroke. Chapter 92. Neuropsychopharmacology: The Generation of progress. Edited by Kenneth L Davis, Dennis Charney, Joseph T Coyle and Charles Nemeroff American College of Neuropsychopharmacology, 2002. pp 1318-1326.

31. Kristian T, Siesjo B. Calcium in ischaemic cell death. *Stroke* 1998;29:705-78.

32. Harraz MM, Dawson TM, Dawson UL. Advances in neuronal cell death—*Stroke* 2008; 39: 286-288.

33. Choi DW. Ischaemia-induced neuronal apoptosis. [Review]. *Current Opinion in Neurobiology* 1996; 6: 667-672

34. Kajstura J, Cheng W, Reiss K et al. Apoptotic and necrotic myocyte cell deaths are independent contributing variables of infarct size in rats. *Laboratory Investigations* 1996; 74:86-107.

35. Saunders J Jr. Death in embryonic systems. *Science* 1988: 154:604-612

36. Yu SW, Andrabu SA, Wang H et al. Apotosis-induced factor mediates poly(adp-ribose)(par) polymer induced cell death. *Proc Nat Acad Sci USA.* 2006;103:18314-18319.

37. Edi er AL, Thompson CB. Death by design: Apotosis, necrosis and autophagy. Curr *Opin Cell Biol 2004*;16:663-669.

38. Eliasson MJ, Sampei K, Mandir AS et al. Poly(adp-ribose) polymerase gene disruption renders mice resistant to cerebral ischaemia. *Nat Med* 1997;3;1089-1095.

39. Bachriecke EH. How death shapes life during development. *Nat Rev Mol Cell Biol* 2002;3:729-787.

40. Lammie GA. Pathology of small vessel stroke. *Brit Med Bulletin* 2000; 56(2):206-306.

41. Fisher CM. Pathological observation in hypertension and cerebral haemorrhage. *J Neuropathol Exp Neurol* 1971; 30: 536-50.

42. Fisher CM. Lacunar infarcts-a review. *Cerebrovas Dis* 1991; 1: 311-20.

43. van Sweiten JC, van der Hout, JH, van Ketel BA et al. Periventricular lesions in the white matter on MRI in the elderly; morphometric correlates with arteriosclerosis and dilated perivascular spaces. *Brain* 1991a; 114: 761-774.

44. van Sweiten JC, Geyskes GG, Derix M et al. Hypertension in the elderly is associated with white matter lesions and cognitive decline. *Ann Neurol* 1991b; 30: 825-830.

45. Klatzo I. Pathophysiological aspects of brain oedema. *Acta Neuropathol* 1987:72(3):236-9.

46. Kunelberg HK. Current concepts of brain oedema. Review of laboratory investigations. *JNeurosurg* 1995:83(6): 1051-9 (abstract).

47. Hemphill JC, Seal MF, Gress DR. In Braunwald & Fauce AS, Kasper DL, Hauser SL, Longo DL, Jameson JL. Editors. *Harrison's Principles of Internal Medicine.* 15th ed. New York. McGraw Hill,2001: 2491-8.

48. Gasche Y, Copin JC. Blood brain barrier, pathophysiology and ischaemic brain oedema. *Ann Fr Anesth Reanim* 2003;22(4):312-9 (abstract).

49. Hart RG, Easton JD. Haemorrhagic infarcts. *Stroke* 1986;17(4):586-589.

50. Paciaroni M, Bogousslavsky J, Levine SR. Haemorrhagic transformation of ischaemic stroke. Med Link. http//:www.medlink.com/medlink.content.asp. retrieved on 4.2.2013.

51. Choi PMC, Ly JV, Sri Kanth V et al. Differentiating between haemorrhagic infarct and parenchymatous intracerebral haemorrhage. *Radiol Res Pract* Vol2012.(2012) Article IDDoi. 10.1155/2012/475497.

52. Brott T, Broderick J, Kothari R. et al. Early haemorrhagic growth in patients with intracerebral haemorrhage. *Stroke* 1997; 28: 1-5.

53. Qureshi AI, Tuhrim S, Broderick JB et al, Spontaneous intracerebral haemorrhage. *N Engl J Med* 2001; 344(19): 1450-60.

54. Chakravathy A, Shivane A. Pathology of intracerebral haemorrhage. *ACNR* 2008;8:20-21.

55. Butcher KS, Baird T, MacGregor I et al. Perihaematomal oedema in primary cerebral haemorrhage is plasma derived. *Stroke* 2004;35:1879-1885.

56. Weller RO. Symposium on hypertension in the elderly. Vascular pathology in hypertension. *Age Ageing* 1979;8 (2):99-103.

57. Anim JT. Cerebral microaneurysms in a Ghanian adult population. An Autopsy study. *Athersclerosis*. 1985;54(1):37-42.

58. Cole FM, Yaks PO. The occurrence and significance of intracerebral microaneurysms. *J Path Bact* 1967;93:393-411.

59. Pezzini A, Del Zotto E, Volonghi I et al. Cerebral amyloid angiopathy: a common cause of cerebral haemorrhage. *Curr Med Clin* 2009;16(20): 498-513.

60. Rensink AA, de Waal RM, Kremer B, Verbeek MM. Pathogensis of cerebral amyloid angiopathy. *Brain Res Brain Res Rev* 2003;43(2):207-23 (abstract).

61. Itoh Y, Yamada M. Cerebral amyloid angiopathy in the elderly: the clinic-pathological features, pathogenesis and risk factors. *J Med Den Sci* 1997;44(1):11-9 (abstract).

62. Vinters HV, Gilbert JT. Cerebral amyloid angiopathy: incidence, complications in the aging brain. ii. The distribution of amyloid vascular changes. *Stroke* 1983;14:924-8.

63. Itoh Y, Yamada M, Hayakawa H et al. Cerebral amyloid angiopathy: a significant cause of cerebellar as well as lobar cerebral haemorrhage in the elderly. *J Neuro Sci* 1995;116(2):135-141.

64. Vinters HV. Cerebral amyloid angiopathy. A critical review. *Stroke* 1987;18:311

65. Blistein MK, Tung GA. MRI of cerebral microhaemorrhages. *AJR Am J Roentgenol* 2007;189(3):720-3.

66. Chen YU, Gurol ME, Rosand J et al. Progression of white matter lesions and haemorrhages in cerebral amyloid angiopathy. *NeuroSci* 2006;67(1):83-7.

67. Ellis RJ; Olickney M, Thal LJ et al. Cerebral amyloid angiopathy in the brains of patients with Alzheimer's disease: CERAD experience. Part XV. *Neurology* 1996;46(6): 1592-6.

68. Arvanitakis Z, Leurgans SE, Wang Z et al. Cerebral amyloid pathology and cognitive domains in older persons. *Ann Neurol* 2011;69(2):320-7 (abstract).

69. Smith EE, Greenberg SM. Clinical diagnosis of cerebral amyloid angiopathy: validation of the Boston Criteria. *Curr Athero Rep.* 2003; 5: 60-266.

5

CLINICAL MANIFESTATIONS AND NEUROLOGICAL SYNDROMES WITH CEREBRAL INFARCTION-ANTERIOR CIRCULATION

Cerebral infarction can be classified into lacunar, territorial and watershed infarctions. The territorial infarction in turn is subdivided into cortical and subcortical. The watershed infarction is subdivided into cortical and internal. The clinical manifestations are divided according to the vascular territories involved, anterior (carotid) circulation and posterior (vertebrobasilar) circulation. The latter are described in Chapter 6. Fig. 5.1 shows the internal carotid, vertebrobasilar systems and the circle of Willis.

I. Lacunar Infarction

Lacunar infarctions are small infarctions that lie in the deeper non-cortical parts of the cerebrum, brain stem and cerebellum and result from occlusion of the penetrating branches of the large cerebral arteries namely, middle cerebral, posterior cerebral and less commonly anterior cerebral and vertebral arteries. Lacunar infarctions range in size from large (1.5-2.0 cms) to small (3-4 mms). About 25% of ischaemic strokes are caused by lacunal infarcts. According to Fisher[1] and Mohr[2] lacunae result from occlusion of a single penetrating artery which is less than 2 mm in maximal diameter. They are not usually detected by CT scan and conventional MRI may not identify the acute lacunar infarction related to the clinical symptoms. Small acute lacunar infarcts have been shown to be detected by MR diffusion—weighted imaging (DWI). The common lacunar sites are the lenticular nuclei (65%), pons (34%), thalamus (32%), and the internal capsule (posterior limb and corona radiata) (27%)[3].

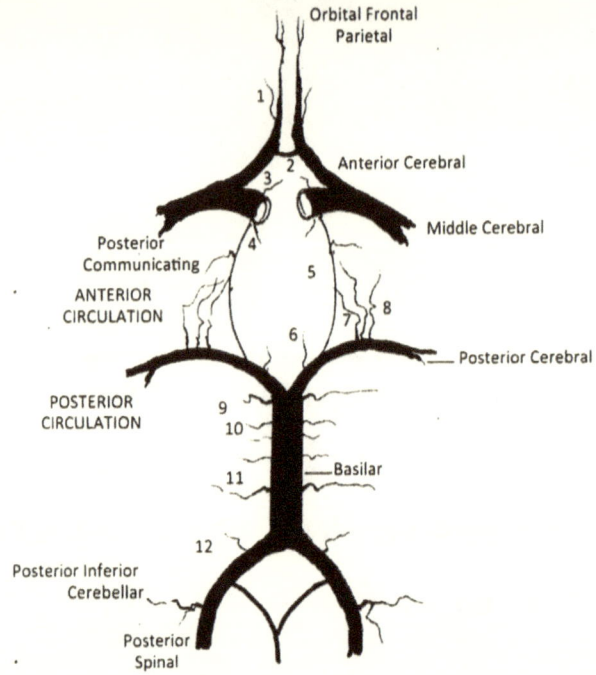

Fig.5.1. Schematic drawing of the Internal carotid/Vertebro-basilar systems and Circle of Willis. The branches are:1. Huebner; 2. Anterior communicating; 3. Ophthalmic; 4. Anterior choroidal; 5. Polar; 6. Thalamic-subthalmic; 7. Thalamo-geniculate; 8. Posterior choroidal; 9. Superior cerebellar; 10. Pontine; 11. Anterior inferior cerebellar.

The proposed mechanisms include lipohyalinosis, microatheroma, vasospasm, reduced cerebral blood flow and endothelial dysfunction. Wassels et al[4] investigating 73 patients with a classical lacunar syndrome found that more than one-third had an embolic stroke pattern with more than one lesion on the DWI and about one-sixth had multiple lesions in different vascular territories. Patients with subcortical infarcts may be seen with cortical lesions and multiple deep lesions on DWI suggesting an embolic etiology[5,6]. Extracranial atherosclerosis or cardioembolic source have been found with lacunar infarcts although this more often seen with cortical infarction[7]. These findings highlight the importance of including a carotid ultrasound, echocardiography, and cardiac monitoring for atrial fibrillation as part of usual evaluation in patients presenting with a lacunar syndrome.

Fisher[8] in 1991 listed more than 70 types of lacunar syndromes with different signs and symptoms. However five classic syndromes, namely pure motor hemiparesis, pure sensory stroke, sensori-motor stroke, ataxic hemiparesis and clumsy hand-dysarthria have been recognised. Table 5.1 summarises the the different characteristics of these syndromes.

Table 5.1 Showing the different characteristics in the classic lacunar syndromes

Syndrome	Pure motor hemiparesis	Pure sensory stroke	Mixed sensory stroke	Ataxic hemiparesis	Clumpsy hand dysarthria
Location sites	corona radiata, IC (genu and posterior limb) pons, medullary pyramid	thalamus, rarely IC corona radiata pons, brain stem	thalamus, IC, caudate, putamen, lateral pons	corona radiata, thalamus, IC lentiform nucleus and pons	corona radiata upper paramedian part of pons, IC anterior limb
Clinical	onset stuttering symptoms, dysarthria, paralysis of face, arm, leg	persistent or transient numbness, hemi-anaesthesia, paraesthetic	motor and sensory symptons	crural paresis & homolateral ataxia incordination out proportion to weakness	facial weakness dysphagia, mild weakness, clumsiness of hand
Other causes	subdural haematoma cerebral diorders	small haemorrhage	haemorrhage	haemorrhages tumours	pontine and putaminal haemorrhages
Prognosis	depends on severity	sensory symptoms subside, in some central poststroke pain	depends on severity	weakness improves, ataxia persists	favourable

Information sources: Kim[9], Arboix etal[10], Nagaratnam et al[11], Arboix et al[12]

Lacunar stroke results from occlusion of the perforating artery and accounts for about 25% of all ischaemic strokes[13]. Hypertension and diabetes mellitus are the major risk factors. In the short term they have a favourable prognosis with reduced functional disability and low mortality but in the long term are at risk of recurrence and dementia[14]. Antiplatelet drugs and risk modification are the main strategies in the secondary prevention of lacunar stroke prevention[13,14].

II. Territorial infarction

Territorial infarction can be cortical or subcortical. Cortical territorial infarction involves the superficial vascular territory of the main cerebral arteries, namely anterior cerebral artery (ACA), middle cerebral artery (MCA) and posterior cerebral artery (PCA). Subcortical territorial infarcts occur in the internal border zones between ACA, MCA, PCA and the areas supplied by lenticulostriate, anterior choroidal and the Huebner (medial striate) arteries.

The mechanisms include large artery atherosclerosis (artery to artery embolism), low flow and cardioembolism. Large artery embolism accounts for about 30% of all ischaemic strokes and cardio-embolic stroke accounts for about 25-35% of all ischaemic strokes. The potential cardioembolic sources with a high risk are atrial fibrillation, infective endocarditis, myxoma, rheumatic mitral stenosis and regurgitation and prosthetic valves[13].

ANTERIOR CIRCULATION

Infarction in the territory of the internal carotid artery (ICA)

The stroke patterns in infarction in the territory of the ICA have been categorized as i. territorial, ii. subcortical, iii. border-zone, iv. disseminated lesions in distal cortical regions and v. embolic. In iv and v fragmented emboli or multiple microemboli occur in small vessels[16] irrespective of the degree of stenosis [17].

Incidence and frequency

Territorial stroke occurred in 47.6% of patients with ICA occlusion[17]. Territorial infarcts are closely associated with border zone infarction[17,18].

Pathogenesis

There are two main mechanisms of stroke in ICA occlusive disease namely embolism and low flow[19]. Unilateral symptomatic atherothrombotic occlusion of the ICA are more likely to be cortical or large subcortical infarcts[20]. A large hemispheric infarction with moderate ICA stenosis may result from a large embolism and or inadequate collateral supply. The stroke pattern in ICA occlusive disease is dependant not only on the degree of stenosis as seen in DW MRI[17] but also in the presence of limited circle of Willis anastomosis[21]. In patients with ICA obstruction the Circle of Willis is an important collateral pathway for adequate cerebral blood flow[22]. A non-functional pathway in the circle of Willis in patients with severe ICA occlusive disease is strongly associated with ischaemic stroke[21,23]. A complete Circle of Willis is an anatomical predisposition for little or no neurological deficits in patients with ICA obstruction[23].

Multiple embolic lesions are common feature of cerebral ischaemia with high grade ICA stenosis. Haemodynamic zone patterns were seen in 31.6% of patients with high grade stenosis and 50% with subtotal stenosis. Territorial infarction pattern was seen in 47.6% of the patients with ICA occlusion[17]. Internal water shed infarction was associated with higher degree of stenosis [25].

INFARCTION IN THE TERRITORY OF THE
ANTERIOR CEREBRAL ARTERY (ACA)

Incidence prevalence.

Infarction in the territory of the ACA accounts for 0.63% [26,27], 1.3% [28] and 1. 8% [29]of all ischaemic strokes.

Pathogenesis

The rarity of the ACA infarction is attributable to the distinctive features of the haemodynamics of the anatomy of the arterial tree[26]. A number of mechanisms are involved i. artery-to-artery embolism from iCA occlusion, cardioemboli[26,27], isolated ACA dissection[27], propagation of thrombus from an occluded ICA and atheromatous changes with secondary thrombosis[26]. The assumed causes of ACA infarction are large vessel disease and embolism (cardiogenic and ICA-ACA embolism). Atherosclerosis is the most important factor in stroke etiology[30] although others have found cardioembolism to be more important[29].

Clinical features

ACA infarction is associated with several clinical features which are more frequent than that seen in patients with MCA and PCA infarctions. Based on clinico-radiological analysis Kumral et al[28] described three clinical patterns depending on the side of the lesion. Those with left-sided infarction had mutism, transcortical motor aphasia and hemiparesis with left leg predominant. Those with right-sided lesion had acute confusional state, motor hemineglect and hemiparesis and those with bilateral involvement presented with akinetic mutism, and severe speech dysfunction. According to them ACA infarction may have similar features to MCA infarction but callosal syndromes and frontal dysfunction may help in the differential diagnosis.

Nagaratnam et al[31] described two groups of patients with ACA infarction. One the para-central lobule group was characterized by contralateral motor weakness, leg more than arm. The paracentral lobule comprises both sensory and motor areas. The second group involving the motor and supplementary motor areas (SMA) had extrapyramidal symptoms apart from the contralateral weakness. The paracentral lobule was said to be involved in 4% of cases with ACA territory infarction, whereas it was associated with the neighbouring areas in 68%, the SMA alone in 6% and in 72% with associated lesions elsewhere[32]. Some of the more important symptoms of ACA infarction are shown in Table 5.2

Table 5.2. Anterior cerebral artery infarction symptoms

Akinetc mutism

Motor dysfunction

Sensory deficit

Extrapyramidal symptoms

Callosal syndromes

Neglect

Language dysfunction

Frontal symptoms

Gait apraxia

Incontinence

Other motor phenomena

i. Akinetic mutism (AM)

AM, abulia and apathy are terms that are said to describe behavioural abnormalities relating to reduced activity and slowness. These clinical states may be a continuum of reduced behaviour and AM may be an extreme form[33]. The clinical picture of AM is associated with different aetiologies and pathologies and they correspond more closely to the functional anatomy of the brain affected rather than the pathology[34].

Unilateral and bilateral infarction in the territory of the anterior cerebral artery is a common cause of mutism with or without akinesia[35,36]. AM has been reported following unilateral infarction involving either the left or right ACA infarction[31,35]. In a study of ten patients with ACA infarction with involvement of the cingulate gyrus six had AM, in four of them the lesion was on the right side and in the remaining two the left. Unilateral lesions are said to give rise to transient AM but prolonged AM lasting for four weeks or more had been reported[31] reduction of spontaneous activity[36]. Depending on the clinical picture AM has been divided into two types based on the anatomic location. One is known as 'hyperpathic' AM and is associated with bilateral frontal damage and the other described as 'apathetic' AM or 'somnolent' mutism and is related to the mesencephalic region[38].

ii. Motor dysfunction and sensory deficits

Motor dysfunction was the most common symptom with motor weakness on the contralateral side of leg[31] and related to SMA and paracentral lobule involvement[30]. Unilateral involvement of the ACA distal to the anterior communicating artery will give rise to contralateral sensorimotor deficits mostly affecting the lower extremity with sparing of the face and hand, frontal lobe symptoms, personality changes contralateral grasp reflex, abulia and motor aphasia. Bilateral occlusion will cause weakness of both lower limbs with sparing of face and hands.

iii. Extrapyramidal symptoms

Bradykinesia, hypokinesia and hypometria with lack of spontaneous gestures and poverty of facial expression occurs[32,39,40,41]. Speech spontaniety is reduced and marked decrease in voice volume were seen irrespective of side of lesion[31]. These patients show involvement of the motor, SMA, prefrontal and parts of the anterior cingulate gyrus and of the sensory cortex[31]. The anterior cingulate gyrus is functionally similar to the SMA and the SMA has afferent and efferent connections with the cingulate gyrus[42]. In a study of nine patients with ACA infarction 3 had asterexis, 5 hemiparkisonism (tremor, rigidity, hypokinesia) and one with both[43]. Parkinonism was related to relatively large lesions involving the SMA and astrexis with small lesions in the prefrontal area.

iv. Language dysfunction

Reduced speech spontaneity, mutism and decrease of voice volume may occur irrespective of the side of the lesion and these symptoms are part of generalsed psycho motor slowing. Language dysfunction with characteristics of transcortical motor aphasia has been reported[28,31]. A pragmatic communicative disorder with difficulty in attuning the train of thought to keep with the conversation and difficulty in controlling speech output was seen in a patient with ACA infarction of the non-dominant hemisphere [40].

v. Callosal disconnection syndromes

The corpus callosum connects the two hemispheres and mediates interconnections between a large number of central processing areas in each hemisphere. The other two interconnecting structures are the anterior and hippocampal or posterior commisures. A variety of deficits in interhemispheric communication have been demonstrated following surgical division of the cerebral commissures and have been described as 'syndromes of brain bisection', or 'syndromes of the cerebral commissures[44]. They have also been described as 'the anterior cerebral artery syndrome'[45].

Intermanual conflict is a dissociative phenomenon in which one hand acts at cross purposes to the other for example when one hand is buttoning the shirt the other hand comes right behind it undoing the buttons. For the alien hand to be persistent will depend on mesial frontal cortical dysfunction[46,47]. Other disconnection callosal syndromes include, unilateral verbal anosmia, double hemianopia, unilateral (left) apraxia of hand, unilateral constructional apraxia, unilateral anomia and. spatial acalculia[44].

vi. Frontal lobe dysfunction

Neurological findings with frontal lobe involvement include abnormal reflexes (the most significant are grasp reflex, the groping reflex, the snout and sucking reflexes), abnormal gait and changes in sphincter control. There is inability to walk, the steps are short without festination, loss of balance with retropulsion[48]. Bilateral involvement of the mesial aspect of the frontal lobe is associated with disturbance of sphincteric control and the patient showing little concern about urinating or even defeacating in socially unacceptable places[48].

INFARCTION IN THE TERRITORY OF THE MIDDLE CEREBRAL ARTERY

Incidence and frequency

MCA infarction increases with age and the highest incidence is in the seventh and eight decades of life[49]. Most strokes occur in the territory of the middle cerebral artery. The frequency of MCA stroke is reported to be more than 80 per 100,000[50]. Usually occlusion is embolic in nature and thrombotic occlusion of the small and large vessels is widely accepted as the primary etiology of strokes in general.

Lateralization of brain function

The two cerebral hemispheres are not equivalent and have different function. Between 70-95% of the population have left hemispheric dominance and includes people who could be considered as left—handed. About 95% of right-handed individuals have left hemisphere dominance for language and is dominant by virtue of of possession of language centers.

I. Left dominant hemisphere

Occlusion at segment M1 will give rise to contralateral hemiplegia, affecting face, arm and leg, hemisensory loss, homonymous hemianopia and if the dominant hemisphere is involved global aphasia.

Post-stroke language disorders

These include aphasia, alexia, agraphia and acalculia[51].

i. Aphasia

Aphasia occurs in 20% or more of patients after stroke[52] and is the most common language disorder among older people. Aphasias may be categorized as perisylvian aphasias (Broca's, Wernicke's conduction and global), non-perisylvian aphasias (anomic, transcortical motor, transcortical sensory, transcortical mixed), other specific language syndromes (pure word deafness, alexia with or without agraphia, aphemia), and subcortical aphasic syndromes and defined by the anatomy of the lesion[51].

Broca's aphasia

Broca's area is situated just above the sylvian fissure anterior to the face area of the motor cortex involving the posterior inferior frontal region[53]. It is characterised by a speech output which is laboured and slow. Articulatory agility is impaired so are repetition and word—fnding. Auditory comprehension is good.

Wernicke's aphasia

Wernicke's aphasia is characterized by fluent verbal output and almost always associated with neologisms and paraphasias. The significant finding is the striking disturbance of comprehension and a corresponding disorder of repetition. Naming is almost always disturbed. It is seen with left superior posterior temporal lesion [53]. The common cause of Wernicke's aphasia with cerebral infarction is embolism with cardiac 40% and large vessel atherosclerotic from the carotids 16% [54].

Conduction aphasia

Conduction aphasia is characterized with severe breakdown in repetition, a relatively normal comprehension and verbal output fluent. In conduction aphasia the comprehension is better than repetition compared to Wernicke's aphasia and differs from Broca's in that verbal output is fluent. The arcuate fasciculus which is said to play an important role in repetition has been re-examined with the use of neuroimaging techniques and the understanding that conduction aphasia is a disconnection syndrome has been challenged[55]. The pathology usually involves the area beneath the supramarginal gyrus but can occur in cases with cortical damage [55].

Anomic aphasia

One of the major features of anomic aphasia is naming or word finding difficulty. To compensate for this some patients resort to circumlocution[56]. Repetition is intact and reading and writing variable. The lesion is in the temporal parietal area. If the angular gyrus is involved alexia and agraphia can occur.

Transcortical sensory aphasia

In transcortical sensory aphasia the ability to repeat is well preserved with fluent speech but impaired comprehension[57] and inability to name, read or write. The Broca's, Wernicke's and arcuate fasiculus are intact and it occurs with multiple sites along the posterior superior and medial temporal gyri[57].

Trancortical motor aphasia

Repetition is good in transcortical motor aphasia but there is non-fluent output except for ability to echo. Comprehension is relatively well preserved so is confrontational naming. There is little or no paraphasia. The lesion is in the area anterior to Broca's area which cuts off the communication between the frontal perisylvian speech zone and the supplementary motor area [58].

Acute mixed transcortical aphasia (MTA)

MTA is characterized by non-fluent aphasia with impaired comprehension . . . impaired naming and with or without echolalia but with good repetition, reading and writing to dictation without understanding. MTA is rare and has been reported mainly in its chronic form in relation to diffuse brain processes[59,60]. Cortical areas may be involved for instance a single lesion in the left frontoparietal region[61] or two simultaneous but independent lesions one in the precentral cortex and the other in the temporo-occipital areas [62]. Subcortical lesions have been associated with MTA[63]. MTA following infarction of the left putamen has been described [64](Table.5.3).

Table 5.3 summarises the characteristic features of aphasia

Type	Fluency	Comprehension	Repetition
Broca's	non-fluent	good	poor
Wernicke's	fluent	poor	poor
Conduction	fluent	good	poor
Global	non-fluent	poor	poor
Transcortical motor	non-fluent	good	good
Transcortical sensory	fluent	poor	good
Transcortical mixed	non-fluent	poor	good

ii. Subcortical aphasias

Subcortical aphasias have been reported in association with lesions in the internal capsule, basal ganglia, thalamus and periventricular white matter in the left cerebral hemisphere [63, 65,66]. Subcortical syndromes are variable and it is believed there is a specific anatomical basis for most variations[67].

The mechanism of thalamic aphasia is still controversial[68]. Kawahara et al [69]described a case with left-sided haematoma of the medial thalamus with aphasia of the mixed transcortical aphasia type. Weisberg[70] described 5 patients with left-sided thalamic haemorrhage who were aphasic and exhibited mixed sensory and motor features with paraphasias, word finding errors, impaired articulation with intact repetition features consistent with transcortical aphasia. There is a likelihood of a more widespread involvement of the surrounding subcortical and cortical structures in cases of thalamic lesions [71]. The clinical picture however is reasonably consistent. In the early stages there is a partial or complete mutism with various disturbances of language dysfunction, expression, comprehension or both but well preserved repetition[72].

III. Territorial infarction-subcortical
Anterior circulation

i. Internal carotid artery—subcortical
The first branch is the ophthalmic artery which enters the orbit to supply the retina and the optic nerve. Next is the posterior communicating artery. The anterior choroidal artery arises just prior the terminal bifurcation of the internal carotid artery into the middle cerebral and anterior cerebral arteries.

Anterior choroidal artery territory infarction
Infarction in the territory of the anterior choroidal artery (AChA) is uncommon. The AChA territory lies between the striatum laterally and the thalamus posteromedially[73]. It supplies the lateral thalamus, and posterior limb of the internal capsule. Cardioembolism is one of the major cause of anterior choroidal territory infarcts[74]. The syndrome combines the triad of hemiplegia, hemianaesthesia and hemianopia on the contralateral side of the lesion[75,76,77]. Incomplete forms are much more common[75]. Two cases reported by Mohr et al[77] showed hypoasthetic ataxic hemiparesis. Slight disorders of speech may accompany left-sided lesions and left-sided spatial neglect with right—sided lesions [75].

Hupperts et al[78] identified 57 patients with AChA territory infarcts by their posterior capsule location on CT scan. They concluded that the posteror paraventricular corona radiata is within the AChA territory because AChA infarcts appear to involve this area. According to Mohr et al[77] the anterior choroidal artery does not supply the corona radiata and lateral venricular wall.

Pathological crying is not a well accepted manifestation of anterior choroidal artery infarction but it has beren reported in this setting[79,80]. According to Anderson et al[81] pathological crying is a single syndrome with different locations and with differences in clinical presentation. Post stroke pathological crying can be distressing to the patient, results in family and carer stress and interferes with rehabilitation.

ii. Anterior cerebral artery—subcortical
Infarction in the territory of the recurrent artery of Heubner
In 90% of the cases it arises from A2 segment of the anterior cerebral artery. It supplies the anteroinferior portion of the internal capsule and anteromedial part of head of caudate. Infarction involving the artery can be silent. The clinical manifestations include weakness of the contralateral arm and face, dysarthria and hemichorea. Bilateral involvement manifests as akinetic mutism[82].

iii. Middle cerebral artery-subcortical

Infarction in the territories of the lenticulostriate arteries (striatocapsular infarction).

Affected structures include the anterior limb of the internal capsule, head of caudate and the putamen. Donnan et al[83] identified 4 pathophysiological subgroups based on risk factors and angiography, i. cardiac emboli to the origin of the MCA, ii. presumed emboli to the same site and/or involvement of haemodynamic factors resulting from severe extracranial carotid artery occlusive disease, iii. occlusion of the multiple lateral striate arteries due to proximal middle cerebral artery abnormalities and iv. normal angiography where pathogenesis is uncertain. The affected areas correspond to the territories of the lenticulostriate arteries but sometimes extend to the territories of the Heubner and the anterior choroidal arteries [84,85]. The major cause of striatcapsular infarction is supposed to be due to occlusion of the orifices of the lenticulostriate arteries at the level of the M1 segment by atherothrombotic permanent occlusion or embolic transient occlusion[84]. Striatocaspsular infarction is known to have variable neurological manifestations including cortical symptoms[85]. The most common clinical presentation is involvement of the upper limb with cortical symptoms such as dysphasia, neglect or dyspraxia[86].

IV. Watershed infarctions

Watershed infarctions occur in the distal fields of two non-anastamosing arterial systems [87] that is the areas between the cortical supply of the ACA, MCA and PCA (cortical watershed infarction) and the more rostral periventricular and supraventricular white matter of the corona radiata and the centrum semiovale[88]. The corona radiata is the watershed area between deep and superficial arterial systems of the MCA, and the centrum semiovale with the watershed zone between superficial system of the MCA and ACA[88]. Together they are called 'terminal supply infarcts'[84] or 'inner or subcortical watershed infarcts'.

The cortical watershed infarction is characterised by infarction in which the border between the the two main cerebral arteries divide the infarct into two approximately equal parts[89,90]. This is the more common form. Inner watershed infarcts involve the vascular inner border zone where the infarct is divided equally by the border between the deep and superficial perforating arteries[90,91,92]. Inner watershed infarcts can be further divided on their radiological appearances into confluent (large single cigar-shaped infarct along side the lateral ventricle) and partial ('chain-like' or 'rosary—like pattern) infarcts [87]. Non-functional collateral blood flow through anterior communicating artery and posterior communicating artery has been associated with watershed infarcts, both cortical and internal watershed infarction[23,93].

Haemodynamic changes in the distal regions of hemispheric blood supply that is in the border zones between major vascular territories can be caused by haemodynamic significant stenosis of the extracranial ICA[24]. It has been postulated that low flow and emboli co-exist in the border zone infarctions and ICA disease[94]. The mechanisms whereby watershed infarctions develop continue to be debated and a haemodynamic cause is usually assumed. Patients with cortical watershed infarction showed preserved perfusion reserve which appeared secondary to the embolism whereas with deep watershed infarcts showed severe haemodynamic impairment especially in Type A (lesions in the centrum semi ovale above the level of the lateral ventricles)[95,96]. Table 5.4 summarises the clinical manifestations and vascular territories of the three main cerebral arteries.

Table 5.4. Summaries the vascular territories and clinical manifestations

	Vascular territory	Clinical manifestations
Anterior Cerebral Artery	About ¾ of the medial surface of cerebral hemisphere	Contralateral sensori-motor deficits mainly affecting the lower limb, personality changes abulia, mutism, grasp reflex sparing face, apraxia, gait dysfuntion, expressive aphasia (L hemisphere)
Middle Cerebral Artery	The cortical branches supply lateral part of the cerebral hemisphere Deep penetrating arteries-pons, caudate.	contralateral hemiplegia, hemianopia, hemianaesthesia; dominant hemisphere-aphasia non-dominant-apraxia neglect-large ones symptomatic; small asymptomatic unless strategically placed
Posterior Cerebral Artery & vertebro-basilar arteries	Posterior 1/3 covexity of the inferior temporal lobe and posterior limb of internal capsule; mid—brain and thalamus	a number of clinical syndromes: left sided—hemianopia with alexia, visual agnosia right-sided-hallucinations and illusions; Bilateral cortical: severe amnesia, bilateral homonymous hemianopia, visual hallucinations Thalamus: sensory-motor with sensory predominating

Information sources: see text

* Cerebral infarction can be categorized as lacunar, territorial (cortical, subcortical) and watershed (cortical, internal) infarctions.

* Five classic lacunar syndromes include pure motor hemiparesis, pure sensory stroke, sensori-motor stroke, ataxic hemiparesis and clumsy-hand-dysarthria.

* The common lacunar sites are the lenticular nuclei (65%), pons (34%), thalamus (32%), and the internal capsule (posterior limb and corona radiata) (27%)[3].

* A complete Circle of Willis is an anatomical predisposition for little or no neurological deficits in patients with ICA obstruction[23].

* The rarity of the ACA infarction is attributable to the distinctive features of the haemodynamics of the anatomy of the arterial tree[26].

* Clinical manifestations of ACA territory infarction includes contralateral sensori-motor deficits mainly affecting the lower limbs, personality changes, abulia, mutism, grasp reflex and sparing the face.

* MCA infarction increases with age and the highest incidence is in the seventh and eight decades of life.

* Middle cerebral artery territory infarction manifests as contralateral hemiplegia, hemianopia, hemianaesthesia, dominant hemisphere aphasia, and non-dominant—apraxia and agnosia.

* Aphasia occurs in 20% or more of patients after stroke[52] and is the most common language disorder among older people.

* It has been postulated that low flow and emboli co-exist in the border zone infarctions and ICA disease[94].

References

1. Fisher CM. Lacunar strokes and infarcts: a review. *Neurology* 1982; 32: 871-876.
2. Mohr JP. Progress in cerebrovascular disease: lacunes. *Stroke* 1982; 13: 3-11.
3. Dombory ML. Stroke: Clinical course and neurophysiologic mechanisms of recovery. Critical reviews in *Physical and Rehabilitation Medicine* 1991; 2(27): 171-188.
4. Wessels T, Rottger C, Jauss M et al. Identification of embolic stroke patterns by diffusion-weighted MRI in clinically defined lacunar stroke syndromes. *Stroke* 2005; 36: 757-761.
5. Roh JK, Kang DW, Lee SH t al. Significance of acute multiple brain infarction on diffuse-weighted imaging. *Stroke* 2000; 31: 688-694.
6. Caso V, Budak K, Georgrades D et al. Clinical significance of detection of multiple acute brain infarcts in diffusion-weighted MRI. *J Neurol Neurosurg Psychiatry* 2005; 76: 514-518.
7. Lee LJ, Kidwell CS, Alger J et al. Impact on stroke subtype diagnosis of early diffusion-weighted magnetic resonance imaging and magnetic resonane angiography. *Stroke* 2000; 31: 1081-1089.
8. Fisher CM. Lacunar infarcts-a review. *Cardiovasc Dis* 1991; 1: 311-20.
9. Kim JS. Pure sensory stroke: Clinical-radiological correlates of 21 cases. *Stroke* 1992;23:983-987.
10. Arboix A, Garcia-Plata C, Garcia-Eroles L. et al. Clinical study of 99 patients with pure sensory stroke. *J Neurol* 2005;252(2): 156-62 (abstract).
11. Nagaratnam N, Xavier C, Fabian R. Stroke-subtype—ataxic hemiparesis. *Neurorehab Neurol Repair* 1999: 13: 67-71.
12. Arboix A, Bell Y, Garcia-Eroles L. et al. Clinical study of 35 patients with dysarthria-clumsy hand syndrome. *J Neurol Neurosurg Psychiatry* 2004;75(2):231-234.
13. Norriving B. Lacunar infarcts. Ther Umsch 2003;60(9):535-40 (abstract).
14. Arboix A, Marti-Vilalta JL. Lacunar stroke. *Expert Rev Neurother* 2009;9(2):179-96.
15. Hankey GJ, Lees KR. Stroke Manangemet in practice. Harcourt Health Communcations, London NW17BY UK. 2001. p3.
16. Baird AE, Lovblad K, Schaulg G et al. Multiple acute stroke syndrome: marker of embolic disease. *Neurology* 2000; 54: 674-678.
17. Szabo K, Kern R, Guss A et al. Acute stroke patterns in patients with internal carotid artery disease. *Stroke* 2001; 32: 1323-1329.
18. Kang DW, Chu K, Ko SB et al. Lesion patterns and mechanism of ischaemia in internal carotid artery disease. *Arch Neurol* 2002; 59: 1577-1582.
19. Rhodda RA. The arterial patterns with internal carotid disease and cerebral infarcts. *Stroke* 1986; 17: 69-75.

20. Mounier-Vehier F, Leys D, Pruvo JP. Stroke patterns in unilateral atherothrombotic occlusion of the internal carotid artery. *Stroke* 1995; 26: 422-425.

21. Hoksbergen AWJ, Majole CBL, Frans-Jan H et al. Assessment of the collateral function of the circle of Willis. *Am J Neuroradiol* 2003; 24: 456-462.

22. Alpers BJ, Berry RG. Circle of Willis in cerebral vascular disorders. *Arch Neurol* 1963; 8: 398-402.

23. Mull M, Schwarz M., Thron A. Cerebral hemispheric low flow infarcts in arterial occlusive disease:lesion patterns and angiomorphologicval conditions. *Stroke* 1997; 28: 118-123.

24. Hartkamp MJ, van Der GJ, van Everdingen KJ et al. Circle of Willis collateral flow investigated by magnetic resonance angiography. *Stroke* 1999; 30: 2671-2678.

25. Del Seta M, Eliasziw M, Streaflar JY et al. Internal border zone infarction. A marker for severe stenosis in patients with symptomatic internal carotid artery disease. *Stroke* 2000; 31: 631-636.

26. Gacs G, Fox AJ, Barnett HJM et al. Occurrence and mechanisms of occlusion of the anterior cerebral artery. *Stroke* 1993; 14: 952-959.

27. Kazui S, Sawada T, Naritomi H et al. Angiographic evolution of brain infarction limited to the anterior cerebral artery territory. *Stroke* 1993; 24: 549-553.

28. Kumral E, Bayulkem G, Evyapan D, Yunten N. Spectrum of anterior cerebral artery infarction: clinical and MRI findings. *Eur J Neurol* 2002; 9(6): 615-24.

29. Abroix A, Garcia-Eroles I, Seallares N et al. Infarction in the territory of the anterior cerebral artery: Clinical study of 51 patients. *BMC Neurol* 2009; 9:30. Abstract.

30. Kang SY, Kim JS. Anterior cerebral artery infarction: stroke mechanism and clinical-imaging study in 100 patients. *Neurology* 2008; 70(240: 2386-93.

31. Nagaratnam N, Davies D, Chen E. Clinical effects of anterior cerebral artery infarction. *J Stroke Cerebrovasc Dis*. 1998;7:391-397.

32. Hung TP, Ryn SJ. Anterior cerebral syndromes. In: Vinken PJ, Bruyn CW, Klawans HL et al. eds Handbook of clinical neurology. Vol 53. New York:Elsevier,1988: 339-352.

33. Caplan LR, Schmahmann D, Kasi et al. Caudate infarcts. *Arch Neurol* 1990; 47:133-142.

34. Nagaratnam N, Nagaratnam K, Ng K, Diu P. Akinetic mutism following stroke. *J Clin Neurosci* 2004; 11(1): 25-30.

35. Bogousslaksy J, Regli F. Anterior cerebral infarctions: Lausanne Registry. *Arch Neurol* 1990; 47: 144-150.

36. Borggreve F, DeDeynPP, Marien P et al. Bilateral infarction in the anterior cerebral artery territory due to an unusual anomaly of the circle of Willis. *Stroke* 1994; 25: 2297-2298.

37. Meador KJ, Watson RT, Bowers D, Heilman KM. Hypometria with hemispatial and limb motor neglect. *Brain* 1986; 109: 293-305.
38. Segarra JM. Cerebral vascular disease and behaviour:The syndrome of the mesencephalic artery. *Arch Neurol* 1970; 22: 401-418.
39. Nagaratnam N. Post-hemiplegic dystonia following right anterior cerebral artery infarction. *Aust NZ J Med* 1991; 21: 381-383.
40. Gapes L, Nagaratnam N. Occlusion of the right cerebral artery causing language disturbance in a right hander. *J Neurol Rehab* 1989; 3: 101-103.
41. Chamorro A, Marshall RS, Valls-Sole J. Motor behaviour in stroke patients with isolated medial frontal ischaemic infarction. *Stroke* 1997; 28: 1755-60.
42. Damasio AR, Vandstensen GW. Structure and function of the supplementary motor area. *Neurology* 1980; 30: 300-359.
43. Kim JS. Involuntary movements after anterior cerebral artery territory infarction. *Stroke* 2001; 32: 258-261.
44. Bogen JE. The Callosal Syndomes. in Clinical Neuropsychology ed Kenneth M Heilman and Valenstein E. third ed. Oxford University Press, 1993. pp 337-447.
45. Critchley M. The anterior cerebral artery and its syndromes. *Brain* 1930; 120-165.
46. Feinberg TE, Schundler RJ, Flanangan WG, Haben LD. Two alien hand syndromes. *Neurology* 1992; 42:19-24.
47. Starkstein SE, Berthier ML, Fedoro P. et al Anosognosia and major depression in two patients with cerebrovascular lesions. *Neurology* 1990; 40: 1381-1382.
48. Damasio AR, Anderson, SW. The Frontal Lobes. In Clinical Neuropsychology. Ed Kenneth M, Heilman and Valenstein E. 3rd Edition. Oxford University Press, Oxford. 1993. pp 409-460.
49. Slater DI, Curtin SA, Johns JS, Schmidt C. Middle cerebral artery stroke. eMedicine Physical Medicine and Rehabilitation. 2009. *http://emedicine. medscape.com/article/323120overview* accessed on 8/04/2010.
50. Barnett H, Mihr JP, Stein B. et al. Stroke: Pathogenesis, diagnosis and management. 2nd ed London, England. Churchill Livingston. 1992: 360-405.
51. Sinanovic O, Mrkonjic Z, Zukic S. et al. Post-stroke language disorders. *Acta Clin Croat* 2011;50(1):79-94 (abstract).
52. Kertesz A, Sheppard A, Mackenzie R. Localization in transcortical sensory aphasia. *Arch Neurol* 1982; 39: 475-478.
53. Kertesz A. Clinical forms of aphasia. *Acta Neurochir Suppl (Wein)*.1993;56:528 (abstract)
54. Knepper LG, Biller J, Tranel D et al. Etiology of stroke in patients with Wernicke's aphasia. *Stroke* 1989;20:1734-1732.
55. Ardila A. A review of conduction aphasia. *Curr Neurol Neurosci Rep* 2010;10(6) 499-503 (abstract).
56. Goodglass H, Kaplan L, Barres B. The assessment of aphasias and related disorders. (3rd ed) Blatimore. Lippincott, Wilson &Wilkins,2001.

57. Boatman D, Gordon B, Hart J et al. Transcortical sensory aphasiaL revisited and revised. Brain 2000;123(8):1634-1642.

58. Freedman M, Alexander MP, Nasser MA. Anatomic basis of transcortical motor aphasia. *Neurology* 1984;34(4): 409-17.

59. Geschwind N, Fussilo M. Color-naming deficits following posterior cerebral artery infarction. *Arch Neurol* 1996; 15: 137-46.

60. Whitaker H. A case of isolation of language function. In H.Whitaker and HA Whitaker(Eds) Studies in Neurolinguistics Vol. 1 New York "Academic Press pp1-58.

61. Ross ED. Left medial parietal lobe and receptive language functions: mixed transcortical aphasia after left anterior cerebral infarction. *Neurology* 1980; 30: 144-150.

62. Bogousslavsky J, Regli F, Assal G. Acute transcortical mixed aphasia. A carotid occlusion syndrome with pial and watershed infarcts. *Brain* 1988; 11: 631-641.

63. Nagaratnam N, Barnes R. Language dysfunction in white matter lesions without significant hemiparesis. *J Neurologic Rehabil* 1996;10:253-56.

64. Nagaratnam N, Gilhotra JS. Acute mixed cortical aphasia following an infatcion in the left putamen. *Aphasiology* 1998; 12: 489-493.

65. Naesar MA, Alexander MA, Helm-Eastbrocks N et al. Aphasia with predominantly subcortical lesion sites: description of three capsular-putaminal aphasia syndromes. *Arch Neurol* 1982: 39: 2-12.

66. Damasio AR, Damasio H, Rizzo M et al. Aphasia in non-haemorrhagic lesions in the basal ganglia and internal capsule. *Arch Neurol* 1982; 39: 15-20.

67. Alexander MP, Naesar MA, Palumbo CL. Correlations of substantial CT lesion sites aphasia profiles. *Brain* 1987; 110: 961-991.

68. Mohr JP, Watters WC, Duncan GW. Thalamic haemorrhageand aphasia. *Brain Lang* 1975; 2: 3-17.

69. Kawahara N, SatoK, Murak M et al. CT classification of small thalamic haemorrhages and their clinical implications. *Neurology* 1986; 30: 65-72.

70. Weisberg LA. Thalamic haemorrhage: Clinical—CT correlation. *Neurology* 1986; 36: 1382-6.

71. Alexander MIP, LoVerme Jr SR. Aphasia after left hemispheric haemotrrhage. *Neurology* 1980; 30: 193-202.

72. McFarling D, Rothi LJ, Heilman KM. Transcortical aphasia from ischaemic infarcts in the thalamus. Report of two cases. *J Neurol Neurosurg Psychiatry* 1982; 45: 107-112.

73. Takahashi S, Fukasawa H, Ishii K, Sakamoto K. The anterior choroidal artery syndrome. *Neuroradiology* 1994; 36(5): 337-339.

74. Leys D, Mounier-Vehier F, Lavenu I et al. Anterior choroidal territory infarcts: study of presumed mechanism. *Stroke* 1994; 25: 837-842.

75. Decroix JP, Gravelean PH, Masson M, Gambier J. Anterior choroidal artery syndrome. *Brain* 1986; 109(6): 1071-1085.

76. Steegmann AT, Roberts AJ. The syndrome of anterior choroidal artery. *J Amer Assoc* 1935; 104: 1695-1697.

77. Mohr JP, Steinki W, Timsit SG. et al. The anterior choroidal artery does not supply the corona radiata and lateral ventricular wall. *Stroke*;1991; 22: 1502-1507.

78. Hupperts RM, Lodder J, Heuts-Van Rask EP. et al,. Infarcts of the anterior choroidal artery territory:anatomical distribution, clinical syndromes, presentation, pathogenesis and early outcome. *Brain* 1994;117:825-834.

79. Derex L, Ostrowsky K, Nighoghossian N et al. Severe pathological crying after left anterior choroidal artery infarct-reversibility with paroxetine treatment. *Stroke* 1997; 28: 1464-1466.

80. Nagaratnam N, Wong V, Jeyaratnam D. Left anterior choroidal artery infarction and uncontrollable crying. *J Stroke Cerebrovasc Dis* 1998;7(4): 263-264

81. Anderson G, Ingeman-Nielsonm, Vestergaard K et al. Pathoanatomic correlation between poststroke pathological crying and damage to brain areas involved in serotonergic neurotransmission. *Stroke* 1994; 25: 1050-1052.

82. Weerakoddy Y, D'Souza et al. Recurrent artery of Heubner. *http://radiopaedia. org/articles/recurrent-artery-of heubner-1* retreived 20.7.11.

83. Donnan GA, Bladin PF, Berkovic SF et al. The stroke syndrome of striatocapsular infarction. *Brain* 1991; 114A: 51-70.

84. Nakano S, Yokogami K, Ohta H et al. CT defined large subcortical infarcts: correlation oflocation with site of cerebrovascular occlusive disease. *AJNR J Neuroradiol* 1995; 16: 1581-1585.

85. Weiller C, Ringelstein EB, Reiche W, et al. The large striatocapsular infarct: a clinical and pathophysiological entity. *Arch Neurol* 1990; 47: 1086-1091.

86. Jung S, Hwang S-H, Lee B-C. Distinct clinical expressions of striatocapsular infarction according to cortical manifestations. *Eur J Neurol* 2004; 11 (9): 627-633.

87. Momjian-Meyer I, Baron J-C. The pathophsiology of watershed infarction in internal carotid artery disease. *Stroke.* 2005; 36: 567-577.

88. Ringelstein ED, Zenner H, Angelou D. The pathogenesis of strokes from internal carotid artery occlusion: diagnostic and therapeutic implications. *Stroke* 1983; 14: 876-875.

89. Bogousslavsky J, Regli F. Border zone infartions distal to the internal carotid artery occluision.: prognostic implications. *Ann Neurol* 1986; 20: 346-350.

90. Ghika JA, Bogousslavsky J, Regli F. Deep perforators from the carotid system. *Arch Neurol* 1990; 47: 1097-1100.

91. Angelino O, Bozzao L, Fantozzi L et al. Internal borderzone infatrction flowing acute middle cerebral artery occlusion. *Neurology* 1990; 40: 1196-1198.

92. Bladin CF, Chambers BR. Clinical features pathogenesis and computed tomographic characteristics of internal water shed infarctions. *Stroke* 1993;24: 1925-1932.

93. Miralles M, Dolz JL, Cotillus J et al. The role of Circle of Willis in carotid occlusion. assessment with phase contrast MR angiography and transcranial duplex. *Eur J Vasc Endvasc Surg* 1995; 10: 424-450.

94. Caplan LR, Hennerice M. Impaired clearance of emboli (washout) is an important link between hypoperfusion embolism, ischaemic stroke. *Arch Neurol* 1998; 55: 1475-1482.

95. Moriwaki H, Matsumoto M, Hashikawa K. Haemodynamic aspect of cortical water shed infarcts: Assessment of perfusion reserve using iodine ~123~ iodoampetamine SPECT *J Nuclear Med* 1997; 381: 1556-1562.

96. Yong SW, Bang Oh Y, Lee PH, Li WY. Internal and cortical border zone infarction. Clinical and diffusion-weighted imaging features. *Stroke* 2006; 37: 841-**846.**

6

CLINICAL MANIFESTATIONS AND NEUROLOGICAL SYNDROMES- CEREBRAL INFARCTION— POSTERIOR CIRCULATION

POSTERIOR CIRCULATION

Infarction in the territory of the posterior cerebral artery (PCA)

Approximately 13% of all cerebral infarcts occur in the territory of the posterior cerebral artery (PCA)[1]. A number of clinical syndromes have been described with PCA infarction depending on the extent of the lesion and location. Depending on the extent of the involvement of the PCA and its branches the lesions could be located in the inferolateral thalamic territory, paramedian thalamic terrritory, in other mid brain or thalamic territories or in combinations[1] (Fig6.1). Distally it supplies the medial inferior temporal lobe, parahippocampal and hippocampal gyri and the occipital lobe including the calcarine cortex and visual association areas. The infarctions are unilateral sometimes bilateral and are commonly caused by embolism either from the heart or from the atheromatous vertebrobasilar arteries. Patients with PCA infarcts can present with a variety of neurological symptoms.

1. *Acute confusional state.* It is well known that focal lesions involving the cortex [2,3] or solely subcortical[4] in the non-dominant hemisphere and in the territory of the middle cerebral artery can give rise to acute confusional state. Devinsky et al [5] described confusional states following PCA infarction. Millandre et al[1] in their study of 82 patients with PCA infarction found no difference in the frequency of the confusional state (n=24) between left and right-sided lesions.

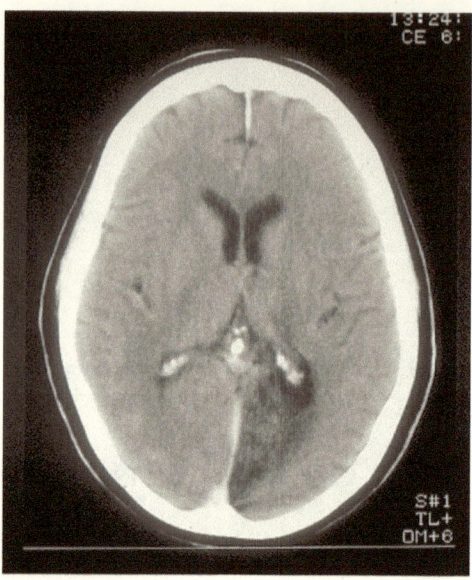

Fig 6.1 CT scan showing inarction in the territory of posterior cerebral
artery ascending into theinferolateral thalamic territory

2. *Visual disturbances.*

Vision loss and field defects

   A lesion in the contralateral occipital lobe can give rise to complete hemianopia,
or with macula sparing if the occipital lobe remains intact from blood supply from
a branch of the MCA. Cortical blindness of varying degree occurs with bilateral
infarction of the occipital lobes depending on the extent of the lesion. Anton's
syndrome is a form of cortical blindness associated with confabulation[6] in which the
patient denies visual impairment. It is caused by damage to the occipital lobe which
extends from the primary visual cortex to the visual association areas.

Visual hallucinations.

   There is a causal relationship between visual hallucinations and the visual field
defect. The right hemisphere seems to have a ceratin degree of predominance for
the occurrence of visual hallucinations[7]. Kolmel [8] however found no predilection for
one hemisphere for patients with complex visual hallucinations experienced in the
hemispheric field.

Visual agnosia.

   Visual agnosias include the inability to recognize objects, faces, and colour.
Object agnosia is the inability to name or indicate the use of an object seen by
spoken or written word or by gesture. The diagnosis requires intact visual acuity
and language function. Prosopagnosia is an inability to recognize faces. It is caused

by bilateral involvement of the occiptotemporal lesions but there has been several reports of damage confined solely to the right hemisphere[9,10]. Another form of aphasia is largely restricted to the naming of colours and according to Damasio and Damasio [11] it is due to involvement of the white matter in the medial aspect of the left cerebral hemispheres just below the corpus callosum and splenium.

Balint's syndrome is characterized by optic ataxia (difficulty in directing the eyes and hands to targets), optic apraxia (inability to voluntarirly guide eye movements/ change to new location of visual fixation.) and simultagnosia (the inability to perceive more than one object at a time). The diagnosis of optic ataxia requires that there is an isolated inability to point accurately to a target under visual guidance, where patients have no difficulty pointing to targets in their own body or garments (somatosensory guidance). It results from bilateral damage to the posterior parietal cortex—parieto-occiptal border zones[12,13]. Optic ataxia has followed unilateral stroke in the parieto-occiptal region but also may be located anteriorly suggesting disruption of the occipto—parieto-frontal bundle[14].

3. Memory loss

That bilateral PCA infarction gives rise to severe amnesia is well known[15]. Acute amnesia following PCA infarction has been associated with damage to the medial temporal structures and in some the splenium is involved[11]. Valenstein et al[16] described a patient with severe amnesia (retrograde and anterograde) following a left sided haemorrhage and MRI showed damage to the splenium, retrospenial cortex and the cingulated bundle. With medial temporal lesions severe amnesia can result only when the hippocampus and amygdala and the subcortical structures are involved[17]. For severe amnesia to occur two systems have to be damaged, one the Papez circuit which involves the hippocampus, fornix, mammillary bodies, mammillo-thalamic tract, inferior thalamus, cingulated gyrus and cingulated bundle. A lesion in the retrospenial cortex underlying cingulated bundle can interrupt the pathway from the hippocampus to the anterior thalamus via the retrosplenial cortex[18]. The other involves anterior temporal cortex, amygdala, dorsomedial thalamus and orbitofrontal cortex [19].

POSTERIOR CEREBRAL ARTERY-SUBCORTICAL

Thalamus and vascular syndromes of the thalamus

The thalamus is a pair of ovoid organs and is situated in the brain stem superior to the hypothalamus and form the lateral walls of the third ventricle. Four regions identified anatomically and functionally are the anterior, posterior, medial and lateral regions which are partially separated from each other by white matter lamina, the internal medullary lamina. Encased within the lamina in the core of the thalamus is the intralaminar nuclei. The thalamus is a relay station subserving both motor and sensory mechanisms[20].

The thalamus derives its blood supply from a number of arteries namely, the polar (tuberothalamic), ii paramedian (thalamic-subthalamic), iii thalamogeniculate and iv. posterior choroidal (Fig 6.1). The polar artery arises from the posterior communicating artery and the other three are from the vertebrobasilar system and are branches of the posterior cerebral artery. The polar artery supplies the anterolateral regions of the thalamus and dorsomedial nucleus partially and the ventro anterior and ventrolateral nuclei[21]. The territory of the polar artery is sometimes taken over unilaterally or bilaterally by the paramedian thalamic artery. The paramedian artery supplies the posterolateral regions, the intralaminar nuclei and dorsomedial nuclei. Pecheron described three possible variations of the paramedian thalamic-mesencephalic arteries, i. small branches arising from both P1 segment, ii. asymmetrical common trunk arising from P1 segment (this variation is called the artery of Pecheron), and iii. from an arterial arcade emanating from an artery bridging the 2 P1 segments[22]. The ventrolateral thalamus which includes the medial geniculate body and portion of the pulvinar is supplied by the thalamogeniculate artery[21]. The posterior choroidal arteries (medial and lateral) supply the the dorsomedial and lateral axis of the thalamus and the anterior nucleus, pulvinar, medial and lateral geniculate bodies[21].

Occlusion of the artery of Pecheron results in bilateral thalamic and mesencephalic infactions. The main symptoms are vertical gaze palsy (65%), memory impairment (58%), confusion (53%) and coma (42%)[23].

Posterior choroidal artery territory infarction
Neau and Bogousslasky [22] studied 10 cases selected from 2,925 stroke patients and 10 published reports. The most common manifestations of lateral posterior choroidal (PChA) territory infarct included homonymous quadrantanopsia with or without hemisensory loss, transcortical aphasia and memory losses. Medial PChA territory is less frequent and eye movement disorders predominate [24].

Thalamogeniculate territory infarction
TGA branches arise in 80% of the hemispheres from P2 segment of the posterior cerebral artery and in 20% from P3 segment [25]. Lesions are located medial to the dorsal third of the posterior limb of the internal capsule. Small lesions affect the lateral thalamus. In a study of 732 stroke patients, 33 had small thalamic infarcts and of them 21 had a lesion confined to the thalamogeniculate artery (TGA) territory [23]. TGA infarcts manifested as pure sensory stroke, ataxic hemiparesis and more rarely hypesthetic—ataxic hemiparesis. Other manifestations include sensori-motor and involuntary movements 19% of their cases developed classical Dejerine—Rousy syndrome [26].

Brainstem strokes

Basilar

The basilar artery is the main blood supply to the brain stem. Brainstem strokes are categorized into a variety of well defined syndromes according to the vascular territory involved.

i. Anterior inferior cerebellar artery territory stroke (AICA)

AICA infarcts are considered rare and underdiagnosed reports of non-fatal cases are rarer still[27,28]. In such infarcts brain stem signs predominate. Vertigo, ataxia, ipsilateral facial weakness and deafness arethe usual clinical manifestations. Unilateral infarcts limited to the AICA territory are usually caused by the occlusion of the AICA itself. Sudden deafness deafness is one of the manifestations of AICA infarcts[29,30] and such deafness may be underdiagnosed. It should be actively sought especially in patients with a risk of stroke who present with other neurological signs[31]. Deafness was seen in 33% of autopsy studies and was present in 3 of the 8 patients with AICA infarcts on MRI[32]. The hearing loss is attributed to involvement of the cochclear nerve or auditory nerve or infarction in the lateral part of the inferior pontine region. The labyrinthine artery usually arises fromm the AICA but it can take its origin from the basilar artery or PICA.

ii. Superior cerebellar artery territory stroke (SCA)

In a study of 21 patients with SCA infarction only two had the classical signs of SCA. Dysmetria, dysdiadochokinesis, dysarthria, ataxia and vertigo were the most common findings[33]. The syndrome of SCA is characterized by loss of pain and temperature on the opposite side of the body, Horner's syndrome with ataxia, weakness and tremor of the upper extremity. Palatal myoclonus had been reported[34].

Vertebral

Lateral medullary syndrome is the most common brainstem stroke. The main blood supply to the lateral medullary area are the direct penetrating arteries from the distal vertebral artery. The posterior inferior cerebellar artery supplies the region in less than third of the cases suggesting that lateral medullary syndrome is only infrequently caused by cerebellar infarction[35]. The patient presents with vertigo, facial pain, nausea, vomiting, headache and imbalance. Signs on the ipsilateral side include loss of sensation to pain and temperature with loss of corneal reflex and facial pain due to involvement of the V nucleus and descending tract. Involvement of the vestibular nucleus causes dizziness and nystagmus. There is inability to stand and walk, swaying and falling with gait ataxia due to involvement of the cerebellum and restiform body. Horner's syndrome is due to involvement of the sympathetic.

On the contralateral side there is loss of pain and temperature on the body due to involvement of the spino-thalamic tract. Dysphagia has been reported in lateral medullary syndrome and although the lesion is unilateral it affects the swallowing bilaterally[36]. Often the lateral and medial medullary syndromes are combined (Babinski and Nageotte syndrome).

   ii. *Medial medullary syndrome* results from involvement of the medullary pyramid which supplied by the anterior spinal artery. It is characterized by hemiplegia, upper and lower limb and sparing of the face with loss of position and vibration sense on the contralateral side. This is accompanied by paralysis of the tongue on the ipsilateral side due to involvement of the hypoglossal nucleus or nerve and lateral leminiscus[36]. In about half the number of cases there is bilateral involvement with flaccid or spastic quadiparesis.

```
┌─────────────────────────────────────────────────────────┐
│                 CLINICAL RELEVANCE—                       │
│   CLINICAL FEATURES-POSTERIOR CIRCULATION SYNDROMES       │
└─────────────────────────────────────────────────────────┘
```

*   Approximately 13% of all cerebral infarcts occur in the territory of the posterior cerebral artery (PCA).
*   A number of clinical syndromes are associated with PCA territory infarction, with left-sided lesions-hemianopia, alexia and visual agnosia with right sided lesions-hallucinations and illusions. with bilateral cortical lesions-severe amnesia, bilateral homonymous hemianopia and visual hallucinations.
*   Anterior syndromes-Thalamus—sensori-motor with sensory predominating.
*   Occlusion of the artery of Pecheron results in bilateral thalamic and mesencephalic infactions. The main symptoms are vertical gaze palsy, memory impairment, confusion and coma[23].
*   Lateral medullary syndrome is the most common brainstem stroke.
*   The main blood supply to the lateral medullary area are the direct penetrating arteries from the distal vertebral artery. The posterior inferior cerebellar artery supplies the region in less than third of the cases.

REFERENCES

1. Millandre L, Brosset C, Botti, Khalil. A study of 82 cerebral infarction in the area of the posterior cerebral arteries. *Rev. Neurologique* 1994; 150: 133-41.
2. Caplan LR, Delvin LD, Pessin MS et al. Lateral thalamic infarcts. *Arch Neurol* 1988; 45(9): 959-64(abstract).
3. Mesalum MM. Attention confusional state and neglect. In Mesalum MM. Principles of behavioural neurology. Philadelphia F.A. Davies 1985.
4. Nagaratnam N, Nagaratnam K. Subcortical origins of acute confusional states. *Eur J Int Med* 1995; 65: 55-8.
5. Devinsky O, Bear D, Volpe BT. Confusional states following posterior cerebral artery infarction. *Arch Neurol* 1988; 45: 160-163.
6. Maddula M, Lutton S, Keegan B. Anton's syndrome due to cerebrovascular disease: a case report. *J Med Case Rep* 2009 3:9028. Doi: 10:4076/1752-1947-3-9028
7. Lhermitte F. 'Utilization behaviour' and its relation to lesions of the frontal lobe. *Brain* 1983; 106: 237-55.
8. Kolmel HW. Complex visual hallucinations in the hemianopic field. *J Neurol Neurosurg Psychiatry* 1985; 48: 21-38.
9. Benton AL. Face recognition. *Cortex* 1990; 26: 497-499.
10. De Renzi Perspective in two patients with CT scan evidence of damage confined to the right hemisphere. *Neuropsychologica* 1986; 24: 385-389.
11. Damasio AR, Damasio AH. The anatomic basis of pure alexia. *Neurology* 1983:33: 573-1583.
12. Damasio AR, Benton AL. Impairment of hand movements under visual guidance. *Neurology* 1979; 29: 170-178.
13. Rondot P, RecondoJ, Durnas RJT. Visuomotor ataxia. *Brain* 1977; 100: 355-370.
14. Nagaratnam N, Grace D, Kalouche H. Optic ataxia following unilateral stroke. *J Neurol Sci* 1998; 55: 204-207.
15. Trillot M, Fisher C, Serclerat P, Schott B. Le syndrome amnesque des ischaemies cerebrales post ericures. *Cortex* 1980; 16: 421-434.
16. Valenstein E, Bowers D, Verfaellie M et al. Retrosplenial amnesia. *Brain* 1987; 16: 421-434.
17. Mishkin M, Spieglen BJ, Saunders RC, Malamut BL. An animal model of global amnesia. In Alzheimer's Disease. A report of progress in research. Aghing Vol 19. Edited by Corkin KL, Davis JH, Growden E, Lisdin and Wurtman RJ. New York: Raven Press pp 235-247. 1982.
18. Mohr JP, Walters WC Duncan GW. Thalamic haemorrhage and aphasia. *Brain Lang* 1975; 20: 3-17.

19. Bauer RM, Tobias B, Valenstein E. Amnesic Disorders. In Clinical Neuropsychology 3rd ed. Edited Heilman KM, and Valenstein E. Oxforf University Press, Oxford pp 561.1996.

20. Herrero MT, Barcia C, Navarro JM. Functional anatomy of the thalamus and basal ganglia. *Childs Nerv Syst* 2002;18(8):386-40 (absttact).

21. Bougousslavasky J, Caplan LR. *Strokes syndromes.* Cambridge Mass: Cambridge University Press,2001.

22. Rangel-Castella L, Gasco J, Thompson B, Salinas P. et al. Paramedian thalamic and mesencephalic infarcts after basilar tip aneurysm coiling: role of the artery of Pecheron. *Neurocirugia* 2009; 20: 288-293.

23. Monet P, Garcia PY, Salion G et al. Bithalamic infarct. Is there an evocative aspect? Radioclinical study. *Rev Neurol(Paris)*. 2009; 165: 178-184.

24. Neau JP, Bogousslasky J. The syndrome of posterior choroidal artery territory infarction. *Ann Neurol* 1996; 39: 779-188.

25. Milsavljevic M, Marinkovic S, Gibo H, Puskas L. The thalamogeniculate perforators of the posterior cerebral artery: The micosurgical anatomy. *Neurosurgery* 1991; 28: 523-530 (abstract).

26. Lee HM, Lee BC, Kang KS et al. Clinical manifestations of thalamogeniculate artery territory infarction. 1996. *http://bbs.neuro.ov* kr/space/ journal/1990/9602003.pdf. accessed 12/04/2010.

27. Fisher CM. Lacunar infarct of the tegmentum of the lower lateral pons. *Arch Neurol* 1984; 46(8): 566-567.

28. Amarenco R. Hauw JJ. Cerebellar infarction in the territory of the anterior inferior cerebellar artery: a clinicopathological study. of 20 casaes. *Brain* 1990; 113(Pt1): 134-155.

29. Amarenco P, Rosingart A, DeWitt LD. et al. Anterior inferior cerebellar infarcts: mechanisms clinical features. *Arch Neurol* 1993; 50(20: 154-181.

30. Nagaratnam N, Mak J, Phan TA,. Kalouche H. Sudden permanent hearing loss following anterior inferior cerebellar artery infarction. *IJCP* 2002; 56: 153-154.

31. Amarenco P, Roulett E, Hommel M et al. Infarction in the territory of the medial branch of the posterior inferior cerebellar artery. *J Neurol Neurosurg Psychiatry* 1990; 53: 731-735.

32. Milandre L, Rumean C, Sangla I et al. Infarction in the territory of the anterior inferior cerebellar artery: Report of 5 caes. *Neuroradiology* 1992; 34(6): 500-503.

33. Erdemoglu AK, Duman T Superior cerebellar artery territory stroke. *Acta Neurol Scand* 1998; 98(8): 283-7.

34. Levine SR, Welch KMA. Superior cerebellar artery infarction and vertebral artery dissection. *Stroke* 1988;19:1431-1434.

35. Sacco RL, Freddo L, Bello JA et al. Wallenberg's lateral medullary syndrome: Clinical—magnetic resonance imaging correlations. *Arch Neurol* 1993; 50(6):609-14 (abstract).

36. Aydogdu I, Ertekin C, Tarla G et al. Dysphagia in lateral medullary infarction (Wallenberg's syndrome). *Stroke* 2001;32:2081-2087.

37. Kumral E, Afsar N, Kirbas D. et al. Spectrum of medial medullary syndrome: clinical and magnetic resonance imaging findings. *J Neurol* 2002;249(1):85-93 (abstract).

7

CLINICAL MANIFESTATIONS AND NEUROLOGICAL SYNDROMES-CEREBRAL HAEMORRHAGE

Stroke includes cerebral infarction, primary intracerebral haemorrhage and subarachnoid haemorrhage. Approximately 15% of stroke is due to primary intracerebral haemorrhage, 5% to subarachnoid haemorrhage and 80-85% to cerebral infarction[1]. Although the mortality had been reduced over the last 10 years yet it still approximates 20%-30% within three months [2].

Primary Intracerebral Haemorrhage (PICH)

Much of the primary intracerebral haemorrhage is due to hypertension and cerebral amyloid angiopathy. Hypertension causes atherosclerosis in both cortical and subcortical arteries. Whereas cerebral amyloid angiopathy affects the vessels of the leptomeninges and cortex with little involvement of the penetrating vessels. The first signs of intracranial haemorrhage are caused by dysfunction at the site of the bleeding and the development of neurological signs will very much depend on the location and extent of the lesion. Epileptic seizures can be an early or late complication of intracerebral haemorrhage and it is much more common with lobar haemorrhage [3]. The more important causes of PICH are chronic hypertension, intracranial aneurysm, amyloid angiopathy, vascular malformation and bleeding diathesis. A study of ICH occurring in hypertensive patients over the age of 80 years showed several differences from that seen in younger people. the The study revealed that thalamic haemorrhage was more frequent in the very elderly and the Glasgow coma scale on admission was a independent predictor of in-hospital mortality in the very elderly group[4].

Small primary intracerebral haemorrhage

Most haemorrhagic strokes are associated with hypertension which causes intracranial small vessel disease known and lipohyalinosis or fibrinoid necrosis. They are common in the middle and early old age. The most common sites of their occurrence are in the brain areas supplied by the deep penetrating arteries such as the basal ganglia (caudate and putamen), thalamus, pons and cerebellum. The haemorrhages are the result of rupture of the end arteries secondary to long standing hypertension. They often produce lacunar syndromes characterised as motor hemiparesis, sensori-motor stroke, ataxic hemiparesis, dysarthria-clumsy hand syndrome and pure sensory stroke[5].

Lobar intracerebral haemorrhage

Intracerebral haemorrhages lobar in location (frontal, parietal and occipital) are designated lobar intracerebral haemorrhages. The incidence increases with age and is the most common cause of ICH in persons 70 years and older[6]. Such patients do not have hypertension[7]. However some investigators have found pre-existing hypertension in 31-55% of patients[8,9] and hypertension is common in primary lobar haemorrhages as in deep pontine and cerebellar haemorrhages[10]. Furthermore they felt that hypertension is a important in the development of lobar haemorrhages as amyloid angiopathy. Cerebral amyloid angiopathy has been regarded as a frequent cause of lobar intracerebral haemorrhages[11] and the particular feature is the infiltration of the cortical vessels (small and medium sized arteries) by amyloid beta protein, a substance found in elderly persons and is a component of senile plaques in patients with Alzheimer's disease. These patients have a greater risk of recurrence. Apolipoprotein E e4 and e2 allelles were found in over half the study cohort and were predictors of recurrent lobar haemorrhages[12].

The symptoms and signs of lobar haemorrhages will depend on the location. In frontal haemorrhages there is weakness of contralateral side, arm more than leg and accompanied by frontal headache. In the parietal, there is hemi—sensory deficit with headache 'temple 'region. Occipital haemorrhage is characterized by ipsilateral eye pain and dense hemianopia. There is fluent dysphasia and poor auditory comprehension in temporal haemorrhage together with pain in the anterior ear [9].

Subrachnoid haemorrhage (SAH)

SAH is often caused by bleeding from either an aneurysm (referred as berry or congenital) or vascular malformation. The aneurysms usually occur at the branching sites of the larger arteries of the circle of Willis. The blood from the ruptured aneurysm spreads through the cerebrospinal fluid around the brain and the spinal cord (Fig.7.1). Vascular malformations usually bleed into the brain and or subarachnoid spaces. Headache occurs in about two-thirds of the patients and is due to the sudden increase in the intracranial pressure. The headache is sudden, extremely severe reaching a maximum in a few seconds, diffuse and poorly localized and could last for a few minutes to hours to weeks. If bleeding is severe death can occur. There is altered level of consciousness from drowsiness to loss of consciousness, restlessness, nausea and vomiting. Few patients may present with acute confusional state[13]. Neck stiffness is seen initially followed by stiffness of the back and legs with photophobia few hours later.

The spread of the blood in the subarachnoid spaces could affect the cranial nerves (cranial nerves III, VI, IX-XII) and adjacent brain structures (hemiparesis, paraparesis and cerebellar signs), the findings depending on the aneurysm characteristics. Distinguishing syndromes are associated with the different aneurysmal locations[14,15] (Table 7.2). Other signs could include subhyaloid haemorrhage, positive Kernig's and Brudsinki's signs. The blood pressure could be raised and there may be fever.

Table.7.1. Common aneurysm locations and neurological findings

Anterior communicating artery(ACoA)	abulia, akinetic mutism visual field defects
Middle cerebral artery(MCA)	hemiparesis, aphasia (L) visual field defects hemisensory loss
Internal carotid-posterior communicating artery junction	ipsilateral III nerve palsy
Basilar artery	bitemporal hemianopia or bilateral III N palsies coma
Vertebral-PCA junction	ataxia, bulbar dysfunction dizziness

Information sources: Types and locations of cerebral aneurysms[14] , Liebeskind[15]

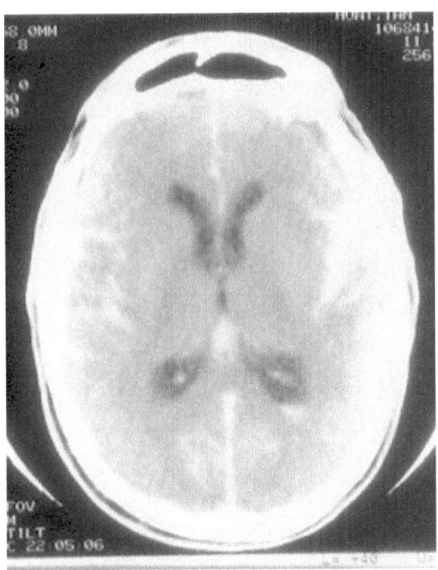

Fig.7.1. CT scan showing subarachnoid haemorrhage

Investigations: CT scan is positive in 85% when performed within 1-2 days. If done early CT is negative and lumbar puncture should be undertaken to look for xanthochromia and is done at least 12 hours after the onset of the headache (to distinguish from traumatic tap).

Treatment: Rebleeding occurs in about 15% of the patients within hours [16]. If no clipping or coiling is done—the risk of bleeding in the first four weeks is about 35-40% [17] and the risk of rebleeding gradually decreases to about 3% a year[18]. Delayed cerebral ischaemia indicates a bad prognosis (usually occurs 4-14 days after the onset) and the mechanism is unclear. It is believed to be due to a combination of factors such as vasoconstriction resulting from the haemorrhage among others[16].

Platelet and coagulation disorders and anticoagulation are common causes of intracerebral haemorrhages in patients presenting to emergency units and so do the abuse of drugs such as amphetamine and cocaine among others and particularly those causing hypertension[19].

SPECIAL TYPES OF INTRACEREBRAL HAEMORRHAGE

1. Putaminal haemorrhage

It is the commonest ICH. It could present with a wide—spectrum of clinical manifestations such as transient neurological deficits (Gunatilleke, 1998)[20], pure motor hemiparesis[21] dysathria-clumsy-hand syndrome, ataxic hemiparesis[5,22] with varying levels of consciousness, neurological deficits, recovery or death. It is usually abrupt in onset with gradual worsening. Global aphasia occurs with a lesion in the dominant hemisphere and hemi-inattention. In large haemorhages there may be a gaze directed towards the side of the lesion (Fig.7.2)

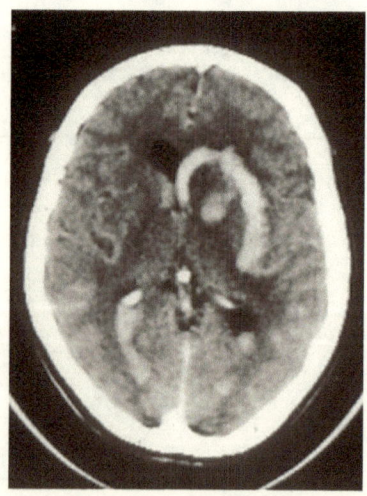

Fig.7.2 CT scan shows basal ganglia haemorrhage

2. Cerebellar haemorrhage

There is a wide spectrum of clinical manifestations from a benign course with little or no deficit to a rapidly fatal case with hydrocephalus and brainstem compression[23]. Nausea, vomiting and vertigo are common symptoms. There is usually a progressive deterioration. About three quarter of the patients with cerebellar haemorrhage have two of the characteristic triad of ipsilateral horizontal gaze palsy, lower motor neurone seventh cranial palsy and appendicular ataxia[24]. Symptoms usually develop during the day when the patient is active. The common symptom is inability to stand or walk. Headache occurred in 36% and vomiting in 44% in one study although they do not exclude ICH[25].

3. Pontine haemorrhage

Presents with bilateral signs, quadriplegia, small unreactive pupils, ocular fixation, ocular bobbing, decerebrate posture, respiratory disturbance and eventual demise[23]. Almost always arises from the paramedian branch of the basilar artery. It often extends into the 4th ventricle with rapid onset of coma and a high mortality. Patients with hemipontine lesions almost all survive (Fig 7.3).

4. Thalamic haemorrhage

Occurs in 13% of intracerebral haemorrhage and 1.4% of all cases of stroke[26]. Usually rapid in onset with vomiting, headache and neurobehavioural disturbances. There is usually an impairment of vertical gaze looking downwards with small sluggish or unreactive pupils. Unilateral sensorimotor deficit with sensory signs predominating. There may be transcortical aphasia or apraxia depending on side of haemorrhage (Fg 7.3).

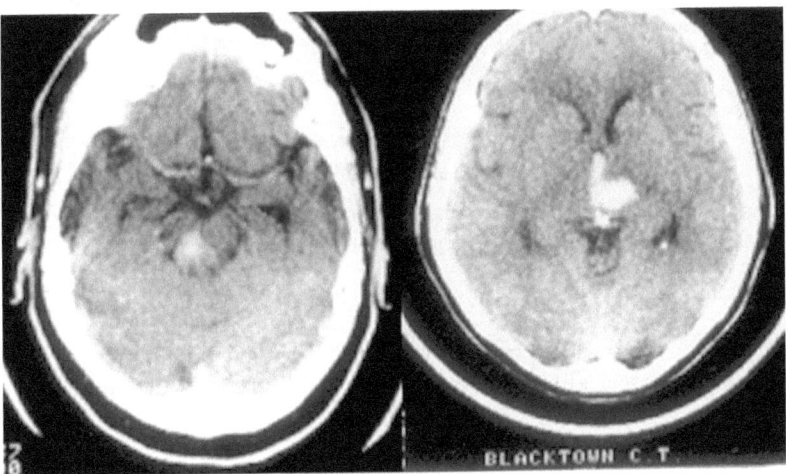

Fig 7.3. CT scans showing (a) pontine haemorhage and (b) thalamic
haemorrhage with bleeding into the third ventricle

5. Caudate haemorrhage

Presents with nausea, vomiting, confusion and disorientation and contralateral hemiparesis and transient hemisensory deficit with a gaze palsy towards the side of the lesion.

6. Medullary haemorrhage

It is rare and the most frequent symptoms at onset are vertigo, dysphagia[23] and sensory symptoms with palatal weakness, nystagmus, cerebellar ataxia, limb weakness and hypoglossal palsy. Less common are Horner's syndrome and facial palsy.

<<Table 7.3. shows the different characteristics with primary intracerebral haemorrhages.

Table.7.3. Primary Intracerebral Haemorrhages

	Deep intracerebral haemorrhage	Lobar intracerebral haemorhage	Subarachnoid haemorrhage
Age	middle age and early	old	young old
Location	basal ganglia, thalamus pons, cerebellum	lobes-frontal, parietal occipital-cortical	Subarachnoid spaces
Risk factors	hypertension	amyloid angiopathy genetic factor	aneurysm, A-V malformations family history (5-20%)
Pathology	small vessel disease— lipohyalinosis fibrinoid necrosis arteriole micro—dissection	cortical vessels infiltrated with amyloid	Congenital defects and degenerative changes
Clinical features	depends on location and size	depends on location and size	depends on location
Prognosis	mortality rate 26% to 56%	mortality rate 26% to 56%	case fatality 32% to 67% 1/3rd of survivors remain independent

Information sources: Vinters,1998[11]; Van Gijn, Renkel,2001[16;] Schieink,1997[27] Hop et al, 2000[28].

* Approximately 15% of stroke is due to primary intracerebral haemorrhage (hypertension and cerebral amyloid angiopathy) and 5% to subarachnoid haemorrhage.
* Small primary intracerebral haemorrhages produce lacunar syndromes.
* Most haemorrhagic strokes are associated with hypertension and small vessel disease are common in the middle and early old age.
* ICH lobar in location are the most common cause of ICH in persons 70 years and older.
* A study of ICH occurring in hypertensive patients over the age of 80 years showed several differences from that seen in younger people.
* Thalamic haemorrhage may be more frequent in the very elderly[4].
* Glasgow coma scale on admission was a independent predictor of in-hospital mortality in the very elderly group[4].
* Platelet and coagulation disorders are common causes of ICH.
* Mortality from ICH approximates 20-30% within 3 months[2].

REFERENCES

1. Bramford J, Sandercock P, Dennis M et al. A prospective study of acute cerebrovascular disease in the community: the Oxfordshire community stroke project 1981-1986. 2. Incidence, case fatality rates and overall outcome at one year of cerebral infarction, primary intracerebral and subarachnoid haemorrhages. *J Neurol Neurosurg Psychiatry* 1990; 53: 16-22

2. Steiner T, Bosel J Options to restrict haematoma expansion after spontaneous intracerebral haemorrhage. *Stroke* 2010; 41: 402-409.

3. Mendelow AD. Spontaneous intracerebral haemorrhage. *J Neurol Neurosurg Psychiatry* 1991; 54: 193-195.

4. Chiquete E, Ruiz-Sandoval MC, Alvarez-Palazuelos LE et al. Hypertensive intracerebral haemorrhage in the very elderly. *Cerebrovasc Dis* 2007;24(2-3):196-201.

5. Kim JS, Lee JH, Lee MC. small lacunar intracerebral haemorrhage. *Stroke* 1994; 25: 1500-1506.

6. Tomonaga M. Cerebral amyloid angiopathy in the elderly. *J Am Geriatr Soc* 1981; 29: 151-157.

7. Massaro AR, Sacco RL, Mohr JP et al. Clinical discrimination of lobar and deep haemorrhages. *Neurology.* 1991;41:1181-1185.

8. Kase CS, Williams JP, Wyatte DA, Mohr JP. Lobar intracerebral hematomas: clinical and CT analysis of 22 cases *Neurology* 1982; Oct 32 (10) 1146-50.

9. Ropper AH, Davis KR. Lobar cerebtral haemorrhages: acute clinical syndromes in 26 cases. *Ann Neurol* 1980; Aug 8 (2): 141-7.

10. Broderick JP, Brott T, Tomsick T et al. The risk of subarachnoid and intracerebral haemorrhages in blacks as compared with whites. *New Eng J Med* 1992; 323: 733-736.

11. Vinters HV. Cerebral amyloid angiopathy. In: Barnett HJM, Mohr JP, Stein BM, Yabsu FM. eds Stroke: Pathophysiology, diagnosis and management. 3rf ed. New York; Churchill, Livingstone,1998.

12. O'Donnell HC, Rosand J, Knudsen K et al. Apo-lipoprotein E genotype and the risk of recurrent lobar intracerebral haemorrhage. *N Engl Med J.* 2000; 342(2): 240-5.

13. Benbadis SR, Sila CA, Cristen RL. Mental status changes and stroke. *J Gen Intern Med* 1994;9:485-7.

14. Types and locations of cerebral aneurysms. *http://www.mcevs.com/sah/saht/pes. html.* retrieved 25/9/2012.

15. Liebeskind DS. Cerebral aneurysms: Clinical presentation.http://emedicine. medscape.com/article/1161518-clinical#0217.retreived 24/09/2012.

16. Van Gijn J, Rinkel GJE. Subarachnoid haemorrhage: diagnosis, causes and management. *Brain* 2001;124(2):249-278.

17. Hijdra A, Vermenlen M, van GijnH. Rerupture of intracranial aneurysms: a clinicoanatomic study. *J Neurosurg* 1987;67:29-33.

18. Winn HR, Richardson AE, Jane JA. The long-term prognosis in untreated cerebral aneurysms.I. The incidence of late haemorrhage in cerebral aneurysm: a ten-year old evaluation of 364 patients. *Ann Neurol* 1977;1:358-70.

19. Wajak JC, Flamm ES. Intracerebral haemorrhage in cocaine use. *Stroke* 1987; 18: 712-715.

20. Gunatilleke S. Rapid resolution of symptoms and signs of intracerebral haemorrhage: case report. *Br Med J* 1998; 316: 1495-1496.

21. Tapia JF, Kase CS, Sawyer JP. Hypertensive putaminal haemorrhage presenting as prime motor hemiparesis. *Stroke* 1983; 14: 50-56.

22. Nagaratnam N, Saravanja D, Chiu K et al. Putaminal haemorrhage and outcome. *Neurorehab Neural Repair* 2001; 15: 53-58.

23. EL-Mitwalli A, Malkoff MD. Intracerebral haemorrhage. Internet *J Emergency Intensive care Med.* 2001, 5. ISSN: 1092-4051.

24. Caplan LR, Mohr JP, Kase CS. Intracerebral haemorrhage. In: Barnett HJM, Mohr JP, Stein BM, and Yatsu F (eds) Stroke pathophysiology, diagnosis and management. New York Churchill Livingstone Chapter 25 Section III Clinical manifestations of stroke 1998; 681-684.

25. Mohr JP, Caplan LR, Melski JW et al. The Havard Cooperative Stroke Registry. *Neurology* (NY) 1978; 28: 754.

26. Arboix A, Rodriquez-Aguilar R, Oliveres M et al. Thalamic haemorrhage vs internal capsule-basal ganglia haemorrhage: clinical profile and predictors of in-hospital mortality. *BMC Neurology* 2007;7:32

27. Schievink W. Genetics of intracranial aneurysms (review). *Neurosurg.* 1997;40:651-62.

28. Hop JW, Rinkel GJ, Algra A. et al. Randomized pilot study of postoperative aspirin in subarachnoid haemorrhage. *Neurology* 2000;54872-81.

8

DIAGNOSIS AND MANAGEMENT
OF STROKE IN THE ELDERLY

Treatment of acute stroke occurs on an ongoing basis beginning in the pre-hospital setting and ending at home after discharge. The sooner the patient gets into hospital the better the chance of survival and recovery. Early identification of signs and treatment are vital. To identify that someone is having a stroke is to remember F.A.S.T. **Face**—Check their FACE. Has the mouth drooped?; **Arms**—Can they lift both ARMS?; **Speech**—Is their SPEECH slurred? Do they underatand you?; Time-TIME is critical. If you see any of these signs, call 000 straight away.

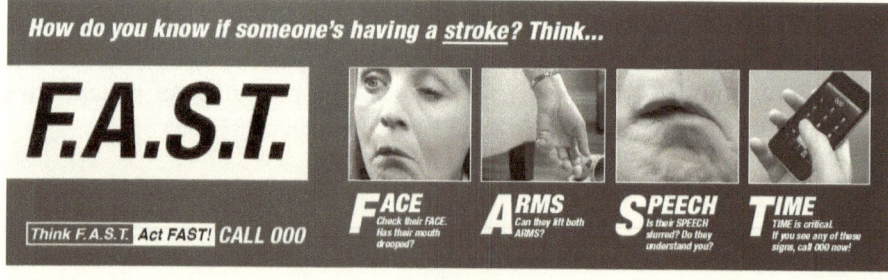

(National Stroke Foundation, reproduced with permission.www.strokefoundation.com.au)

Management of stroke is multifactorial and includes several aspects of care. There is considerable evidence to indicate that stroke care units, critical pathways to process rapidly, identification and evaluation of potential stroke patients and multidisciplinary rehabilitation are associated with improved functional outcome. Timely evaluation and diagnosis is foremost because of the narrow therapeutic window in the treatment of acute ischaemic stroke. Initial assessment involves a history, physical examination, thorough neurological and cardiovascular examinations including diagnostic and cardiac tests. In emergency assessment of a patient suspected of stroke brain imaging is a required component and requisite before any specific therapy[1] Both CT and MRI are used although CT is available in most institutions and hence remains the most applied brain imaging test.

Neuroimaging in Stroke

According to Rowley[2] imaging of patients with acute stroke should be directed towards assessment of i. the parenchyma (detection of intracranial haemorhage) ii. the pipes (identification of intravascular thrombi) and iii. perfusion and penumbra (differentiation of infarcted tissue from salvageable tissue. Imaging provides a guide and this approach facilitates the selection of appropriate therapy and predict clinical outcome[1]. There is now a need to extend the therapeutic window from 3 to more than 6 hours. To do this the following issues have to be addressed, namely the presence of haemorrhage, treatable intravascular thrombus, size of the core and the presence of hypoperfused tissue[3].

Ischaemic infarction can be divided into four stages namely, hyperacute stage (24 hours), acute (after 24 hours) subacute (8-21 days) and chronic (more than 21 days. These findings are related to the time between ischaemia or symptom onset and scanning. Table 8.1 summarises the changes that occur with time in CT and MRI. The use of MRA in combination with MRI +DWI for determining the vascular territory of ischaemic state has a sensitivity of 89-100% and a positive predictive value of 95-100%[8]. In the diagnosis of hyper ischaemic stroke diffusion-weighted MR imaging has a lower interrater variability and greater accuracy[9]. According to Schellinger et al[10] CT sequences can be performed in a few minutes and a combination of MRI sequences in ten minutes. Non-enhanced CT (NECT), CT angiography (CTA) and CT perfusion (CTP) imaging can be used in combination for a quick comprehensive and accurate evaluation of acute stroke[3]. CTA is used to detect thrombi within the intracranial vessels and for evaluation of the carotid and vertebral vessels in the neck and of the arch of the aorta. Gradient-recalled echo(GRE) is better than CTA for detecting distal clot and CTA is better in detecting proximal arterial thrombus[11].

Table 8.1. Infarction in CT and MRI of the brain

CT in Hyperacute stage obscuration of the lentiform nucleus loss of distinction between white and grey matter hyperdense middle cerebral artery sign (Fig 8.1) effacement of the surface sulci (Fig 8.2) hypoattenuation of the insular cortex, 'insular sign'(Fig 8.2)

Acute stage (Fig 8.3) clear demarcation brain oedema mass effect

Subacute stage brain oedema subsides haemorrhagic transformation may occur luxury perfusion

In second and third week hypodense to isodense—'fogging effect'

Chronic stage sharply marginated and well defined ipsilateral ventricle and sulci dilated zone of cystic encephalomalacia and gliosis

MRI

The area of increased MR signal is visualized in

T2 weighted image and in FLAIR mode even in the first 24 hours.

Diffuse weighted image (DWI) will be positive reaching maximum at 7 days

T2DWI—the hyperintensity will be maximum between 7-30 days

Information sources:Moulin et al[4]; Abdulla et al[5]; Becker et al [6], Skriver et al[7]

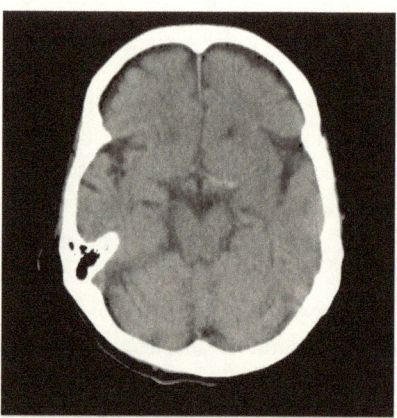

Fig. 8. 1. CT scan showing hyperdense artery in the hyperacute phase

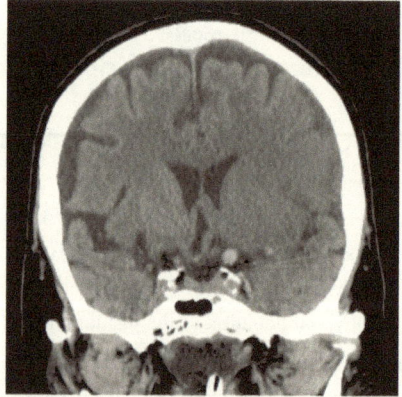

Fig. 8.2. CT scan showing effacement of the surface sulci and hypoattenuation of insular cortex- 'ribbon sign'.

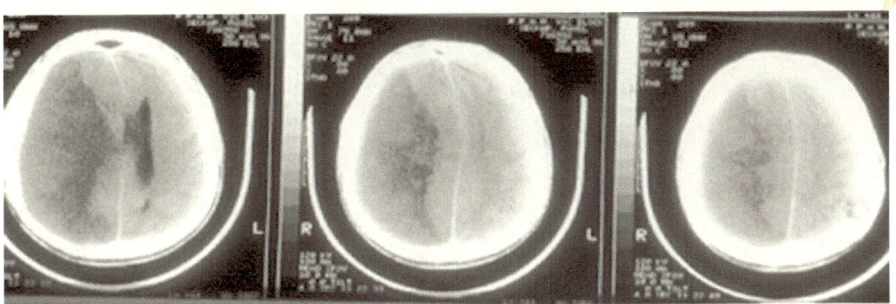

Fig. 8.3. CTscan showing infarction in the territory of the middle cerebral artery, clearly defined, brain oedema and mass effect in the acute phase

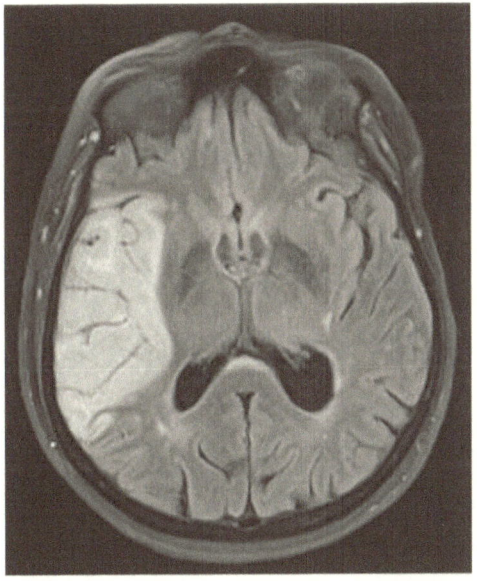

Fig.8.4. MRI—Axial FLAIR—weighted sequence.
In the acute phase—hyperintense on FLAIR

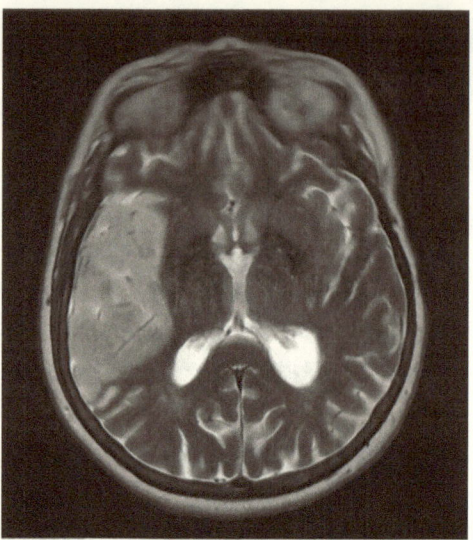

Fig. 8.5. MRI-Axial T2 sequence.
In the acute phase—hyperintense on T2

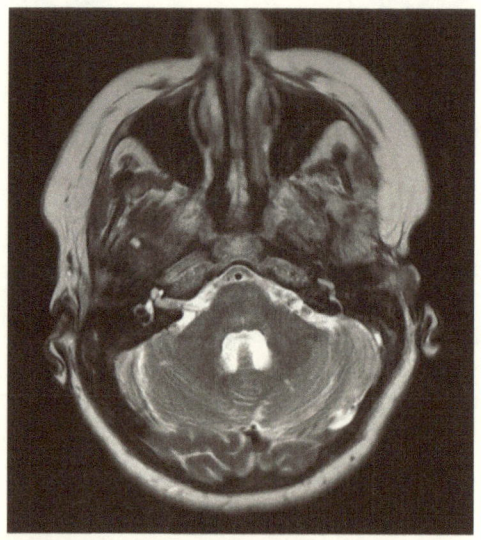

Fig. 8.6. MRI-Acute T2 weighted sequence showing hyperintense thrombus in the horizontal right petrous portion of the right ICA while there is a normal back flow void in the left ICA.

Lacunar infarctions are usually not detected by CT scan and conventional MRI may not identify the acute lacunar infarction related to the clinical symptoms. Small acute lacunar infarcts have been shown to be detected by MR diffusion—weighted imaging (DWI). DWI has demonstrated multiple infarctions in 1 of every 6 patients presenting with classic lacunar syndrome[12]. Extracranial atherosclerosis or cardioembolic source have been found with lacunar infarcts although this is more often seen with cortical infarction. These findings highlight the importance of including a carotid ultrasound, echocardiography, and cardiac monitoring for atrial fibrillation as part of usual evaluation in patients presenting with a lacunar syndrome.

Early Intervention

Early diagnosis is followed by early intervention. Several studies have shown the efficacy of admitting stroke patients to specific stroke care units manned by specially trained staff. In stroke the underlying cause can be either be a haemorrhage or ischaemia and hence the management will vary.

I. Acute Ischaemic stroke(AIS)

Specific

Thrombolytic therapy

Ischaemic stroke results from blocking of the artery by a clot and the aim of treatment is to remove the blockage. The clot can either be broken down (lysis) by pharmacological means or removed by mechanical means (thrombectomy) permitting reperfusion of the ischaemic neurons. Any delay in resumption of blood flow will result in greater damage to the neurons.

Pharmacological thrombolysis involves the use of such agents as tissue plasminogen activator (tPA) or streptokinase. The use of streptokinase has fallen out of favour and three major randomized controlled trials of streptokinase in AIS were curtailed because of safety concerns. The use of tPA however has been supported by results of randomised controlled trials and meta-analysis. The NINDS clinical trials showed the efficacy of tPA in the treatment of patients with AIS and its use has been endorsed by the American Heart Association and the American Academy of Neurology[13]. It is a recommended treatment for AIS within 3 hours of onset provided there are no contraindications and rigid treatment protocol is adhered to[13]. A more recent study by the European Co-operative Acute Stroke Study (ECASS) in 2008 using alteplase in AIS suggested clinical benefit within 3-4.5 hours after the stroke onset. The improved 90-day outcome in patients was comparable to NINDS so were the mortality and cerebral haemorrhage rates but there was a larger number of large parenchymatous bleeds[14]. The ATLANTIS study attempted to increase the therapeutic window from 3 to 5 hours with tPA. The 90 day morbidity was not improved and the mortality and intracranial haemorrhage rates were higher[15]. One study concluded that rt-PA (recombinant tissue plasminogen activator) in patients over 80 years appear to be safe and efficacious and that therapy should not be withheld on basis of age[16]. The more recent data provided by the IST-3 trial confirms the benefit of intravenous rt-PA to patients over the age of 80 years especially when given early and is greatest within 3 hours[17]. The time window remains unclear but data suggest that benefit may extend up to 4.5 hours or beyond to 6 hours in some patients based on individual and combined patients' characteristics[17].

Patients who satisfy the inclusion and exclusion criteria are provided with thrombolysis in stroke care units. rtPA is the treatment of choice for patients who present within 3 hours of the onset of stroke symptoms. Some of the contraindications to thrombolysis with tPA are, severe stroke, seizure at onset, symptoms more than 3 hours or time of onset not known, history of prior stroke with concomitant diabetes, prior stroke within the last 3 months, platelet count < 100,000 per mcL, SBP >185mmHg and DBP >110mmHG and blood glucose <2.8 or > 22 mmol/L[18]. The rate of symptomatic intracerebral haemorrhage in The European Safe Implementaion of Thrombolysis in Stroke Monitoring Study (SITS-MOST) was 7.3% with a calculated mortality rate of 1.9% at 3 months[19]. The Cleveland study reported intracerebral haemorrhage of 22%[20].

Intra-arterial thrombolysis. In intra-arterial thrombolysis the thrombolytic is delivered near the occlusive thrombus through a microcathether and has been found to better the outcome. This has theoretical advantage over intravenous administration and includes local delivery of agent as well reduced systemic effect.

Thrombectomy. In patients with a large vessel AIS due to a large clot it may be less likely to recanalize with the use of tPA. In such situations endovascular mechanical thrombectomy is an option in this subgroup and in those who are unable to receive tpA. High rates of successful recanalization (57.8%) with fewer periprocedural complications in 6.9% were reported by the Multi-MERCI study[21].

Angioplasty and stenting. The availability of self expanding intracranial atherosclerotic stents (SEIS) which can be deployed rapidly and safely has made acute stenting an option in treating AIS. A high degree of technical success (97%) and a 4.6% rate of complications were reported by an NH funded registry[22].

Malignant middle cerebral artery infarction
Incidence is estimated to be less than 1% of all strokes [23].

Clinical features. Malignant MCA infarction is characterized by a rapid progression of neurological deficits with pronounced space occupying effect resulting in transtentorial herniation[24]. Coma terminates in brain death within 2 to 5 days of onset[23]. It is one of the most ravaging forms of ischaemic infarct with a mortality of approximately up to 80% with medical treatment[24].

Symptoms such as disordered sensorium together with neurological decline should alert the clinician to this syndrome in a patient with a large MCA infarct and supported by radiological evidence of cerebral oedema and mass effect. Young patients are particularly prone to mass effect unlike the elderly patient with atrophy that makes them more tolerant to focal infarct-related oedema[23].

Patients with malignant MCA infarction very often have gaze deviation due to involvement of the frontal eye fields together with flaccid hemiplegia[25], hemianaesthesia with global aphasia in dominant hemisphere involvement and severe hemispatial neglect with non-dominant involvement.

Management.

Hemicraniectomy is thought of as an essential life saving measure but there is continuing debate on its appropriateness. The chances of survival may be higher after the operation[25] but mortality and functional outcome is worse in patients especially in those over the age of 60 years[26]. Although observational studies have suggested a reduction in mortality with associated functional gains[27], many clinicians are hesitant to do what they feel or believe is a heroic but potentially a futile procedure except in a few selected patients[28.]

ii General measures

The physiological parameters such as increase in temperature, hypoxia, blood pressure (hyper-/hypotension), glucose levels (hypo/hyperglycaemia), hydration/ nutrition and cardiac arrhythmias in AIS can exacerbate brain damage and worsen outcome[28]. Control of the physiological parameters such as glucose and blood pressure together with intense monitoring has been cited as one of the benefits of acute stroke unit care. Physiological monitoring is an essential part of acute stroke unit care[28].

Hyperglycaemia after acute stroke is associated with poor outcome. Persistent hyperglycaemia more than 155mg/dl is a common observation in acute ischaemic stroke patients and is associated with poorer outcome and higher mortality[29]. However there is no general agreement as to the optimal method of glycaemic control and how intensely the glucose levels should be lowered avoiding the risks of hypogylcaemia[28].

Elevated blood pressures occurred in 80% of the patients with acute stroke on presentation and approximately 30% had a history of hypertension[30]. 60% of the stroke patients are left normotensive due to spontaneous falls in the blood pressures in 4-10 days[31]. Cerebral blood flow is maintained within normal limits by cerebral autoregulation and becomes impaired after acute stroke. Cerebral blood flow becomes dependent on systemic blood pressure and any reduction of the systemic blood pressure will reduce the cerebral blood flow to the ischaemic penumbra. Impaired autoregulation occurs in patients with chronic hypertension and autoregulation occurs at higher blood pressure. This means that antihypertensive therapy may have deleterious effects. The Scandinavian Candessartan Acute Stroke Trial (SCAST) has shown that there is a risk of stroke progression with lowering of blood pressure in the acute phase of stroke[32].

Severe hypertension contributes to brain oedema and increases the risk of haemorhagic transformation. Patients identified for tPA administration must have their blood pressure elevations treated aggressively and in others with ischaemic stroke for minimizing the risk of intracerebral haemorrhage. Two readings should be taken at 5 minutes apart and if the systolic blood pressure (SBP) is 130-230mmHg or diastolic blood pressure (DBP) 105-120mmHg or SBP >230 mmHg or DBP 120-140mmHg in a single reading IV labetolol boluses are employed and when the DBP is more than 140mmHg continuos IV nitroprusside is employed[33].

Temperature. It is recommended that the temperature be maintained normothermic at 36.0-37.0 C with antipyretics and with antibiotics where appropriate. Hyperthermia and hypoxia can exacerbate cerebral oedema.

Hydration/Nutrition. Sustaining nutrition is vital because dehydration or malnutrition will have detrimental effect on stroke recovery. Dehydration is a potential cause of deep vein thrombosis after stroke. It is believed that saline infusion in the first 24 hours may improve cerebral blood flow by preventing drop in arterial blood pressure and dehydration.

Oxygenation. Stroke patients are prone to develop aspiration pneumonia, hypoventilation, atelectasis and pulmonary embolism and are at risk of hypoxia. Hypoxic patients must be given supplemental oxygen if the oxygen saturation is below 95%. However it should not be given to non-hypoxic patients with mild and moderate stroke [34].

Cardiac effects. There is clinical and experimental evidence for neurocardiac links between the insular cortex and its subcortical connections which is the site of cardiac representation[35]. It plays an important role in stroke—related changes. Damage to the cerebral areas results in increased sympathicoadrenal tone causing cardiac myocyte damage and repolarizing ionic shifts giving rise to ECG repolarization changes and arrhythmogenesis[36]. It is suggested that patients with acute stroke should have cardiac monitoring for three days following the event. Those with ECG evidence of ventricular repolarization should have continued monitoring till it is resolved. These patients are at risk of sudden death or stroke extension due to cardiac arrthyhmias[35].

Intracerebral haemorrhage (ICH)

Figures 8.7 and 8.8 shows CT and MRI in acute intracerebral haemorrhage. In intracerebral haemorrhage therapy is largely supportive. It carries a high mortality with a 30 day mortality of approximately 40%. There are many factors that influence the management of ICH, such as haematoma growth, oedema, blood pressure and cerebral perfusion. Other factors being acute hypoxia, fever, increased intracranial pressure among others. Early haematoma growth occurs in 18-38% of the patients within 3 hours of ICH onset[37]. The haematoma volume at presentation with further increase in the volume and development of intraventricular haemorrhage have been shown to be independent predictors of poor outcome and hence early restriction of intracerebral haemorrhage is of paramount importance. In selected patients early treatment with IV haemostasis and minimally invasive surgery may improve mortality and outcome[38].

Recombinant activated Factor VII (rFVII) has been tried to reduce the haematoma growth after ICH. It was reported that treatment with rFVII within 4 hours of the onset limited haematoma growth and improved functional outcome at 90 days. A small phase II trial evaluated a wide range of doses of rFVII found there were no safety concerns[39]. A further study in an international phase III trial is underway.

The American Heart Association and American Stroke Association have set out evidence-based guidelines for treatment of spontaneous intracerebral haemorrhage in adults[40]. Ideally the patient should be in the intensive care unit for monitoring and treatment. Initial treatment includes control of blood pressure (more aggressively compared to patients with ischaemic stroke) bearing in mind that overaggressive treatment[41,42] Increased intracranial pressure is controlled by osmotherapy, controlled hyperventilation and barbiturate coma and ventricular drains in those with or at risk of hydrocephalus[42]. Prophylactic anti-epileptic therapy for patients with ICH may be considered for one month[42]. Patients with cerebellar haemorrhage who show neurological deterioration or have brain stem compression and/or hydrocephalus will require surgical evacuation as soon as possible[43].

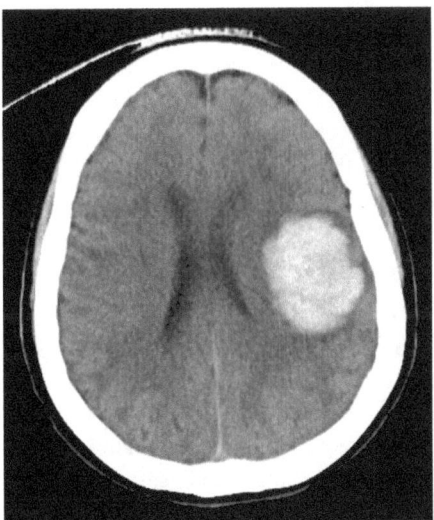

Fig. 8.7. CT scan—showing acute intracerebral haemorrhage

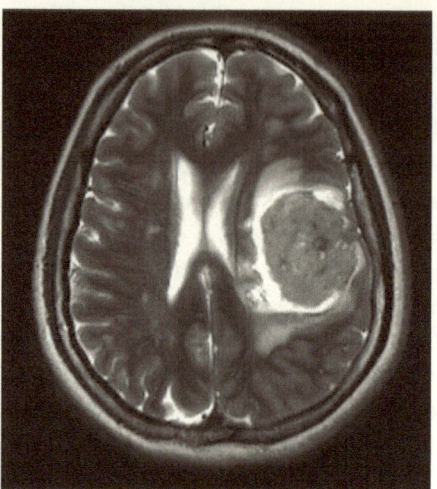

Fig. 8.8. MRI—Axial T2—weighted sequence-acute
intracerebral haemorrhage

iii. Identification of complications

The stroke patient must be closely monitored for neurological and medical complications. Early and late complications are shown in Table 8.2. Prevention of decubitus ulcers begins with thorough skin evaluation at the time of admission. The risk factors include the dependence in mobility, peripheral vascular disease, diabetes, urinary incontinence and lower body mass index [40]. After stroke constipation and fecal impaction are common.

Table 8.2. Complications of stroke-early and late

With 2-3 days—cerebral oedema, increased intracranial pressure, possible trans-tentorial herniation and death; haemorrhagic transformation and seizures Aspiration pneumonia;deep vein thrombosis, urinary tract infection, septicaemia. Late complications-decubitus ulcers, spasticity, contractures. Post-stroke depression

iv. Rehabilitation

The practice in stroke care units is to commence rehabilitation from day one as soon as the condition is stabilized. Rehabilitation assessments should include evaluation of cognitive, communicative skills, physical functioning and psychosocial history and resources[40]. Table.8.3 shows the complications encountered in the rehabilitation unit. Some of the barriers to recovery are severe motor deficit, poor motivation, depression, prior prestroke health, communication problems and perceptual impairment. Several studies have demonstrated the benefits of stroke unit rehabilitation regardless of age and the need for additional therapy in facilitating functional recovery [see Chapter 9].

Table 8.3. Post stroke in rehabilitation unit

Spasticity, spastic dystonia, spasms
Shoulder hand syndrome, shoulder subluxation
Depression, emotionalism, anxiety
Fatigue
Deep vein thrombosis, pulmonary embolism
Post stroke seizures
Falls
Urinary incontinence/retention
Recurrent stroke
Cardiovascular events-acute coronary syndrome,
cardiac failure, arhythmias

Information sources: Dromerick an Reding[44]

v. Prevention of recurrent stroke

The acute hospitalization is focused not only on treatment of the acute stroke but also in identifying risk factors for recurrent stroke. Poststroke outpatient care is largely rehabilitation and prevention of recurrent stroke. The risk factors for stroke include hypertension, diabetes, hyperlipidaemia, diabetes and life style factors such as smoking, alcohol abuse, diet and activity [see Chapter 8].

CLINICAL RELEVANCE—MANAGEMENT OF STROKE

* The primary care physician should recognize the signs and symptoms of stroke, expedite transportation to the correct hospital and early notification of arrival in hospital.

* Computerized tomography (CT) and magnetic resonance (MRI) have virtually revolutionalized diagnostic neurology and neuroradiology.

* The safety and efficacy of intravenous thrombolytic therapy has been highlighted in a number of studies.

* rt-PA (recombinant tissue plasminogen activator) in patients over 80 years appear to be safe and efficacious and that therapy should not be withheld from older people on grounds of age[16].

* The IST-3 trial confirmed the benefit for patients older than 80 years particularly when given early and is greatest within the 3 hour window period[17].

* The chances of survival after hemicraniectomy for malignant MCA infarction may be higher after the operation but mortality and functional outcome is worse in patients especially in those over the age of 60 years 60[25].

* Patient with stroke symptoms and after excluding haemorrhage by CT or MRI should be given aspirin 150-300mg daily as soon as possible.

* An important component of acute stroke care is physiological monitoring and include elevated blood pressure, hyperglycaemia, temperature, oyygenation, hydration/nutrition, and cardiac effects[26].

* Several factors influence the management of ICH such as haematoma growth, oedema, blood pressure and cerebral perfusion.

* It is reported that recombinant activated Factor VII (rFVII) within 4 hours limited haematoma growth and improved functional outcome at 90 days.

* A forceful stroke rehabilitation program is crucial for best functional outcome and elderly stroke patients should not be denied rehabilitation based solely on age.

* After discharge from hospital the basic issues for primary care physician are secondary prevention strategies and patient adhering to post-stroke rehabilitation guidelines.

REFERENCES

1. Srinivasan A, Goyal M, Al Azri F, Lum C. State of the art imaging of acute stroke. *Radiographics* 2006;26 (Suppl 1): S75-95.
2. Rowley HA. The four Ps of acute stroke imaging, parenchyma, pipes, perfusion and penumbra. ANJR. *Am J Neuroradiol.* 2001; 22: 599-600.
3. Latchaw RE, Alberts MJ, Lev MH, Connors JJ, Harbaugh RE, Higashida RT et al. Recommendations for imaging of acute ischaemic stroke. *Stroke* 2009; 40: 3646-3678.
4. Moulin T, Tatu L, Vuillier F, Cattin F. Brain CT scan for acute cerebral infarction: early sign of ischaem, ia. Rev Neurol (Paris) 1999;155(9) 647-55.
5. Abdulla H, Boguslawsky R, Poniatowska R. Hyperacute infarction. Early CT findings. *Med Sci Monit* 2000;6(5):1027-30.
6. Becker H, Desch H, Hacker H, Penez A. CT fogging effect with ischaemic cerebral infarct. *Neuroradiology* 1979;28(4):185-92.
7. Skriver EB, Olsen TC. The transient disappearance of cerebral infarcts on CT scan, the so-called fogging effect. *Neuroradiology* 1981;22(2):61-9.
8. Lee L, Kidnell CS, Algers J. Impact of stroke subtype. Diagnosis of earlyDWMR imaging amd MRA. *Stroke* 2000;31:1183-9.
9. Fiebach JB, Schellinger PD, Jansen O, Meyer M, Wilde P, Bender J et al. CT and diffusion-weighted MR imaging in randomized order:diffusion-weighted imaging results in higher accuracy and lower interater variability in the diagnosis of hyperacute ischaemic stroke. *Stroke* 2002;33:2206-2210.
10. Schellinger PD, Jansen O, Fiebach JB, Pohlers O, Ryssel H, Heiland S. et al. Feasability anf practicality of MR imaging for stroke in the management of hyperacute cerebral ischaemia. *ANJR Am J Neuroradiol.* 2000; 21:1184-1189.
11. Sheikh WS, Gonzal RG, Lev MH. Detection of intracranial thrombus in acute ischaemic stroke by CTA and susceptibility changes on precontrast perfusion MR imaging. Presented at 91st Scientific Assembly and Annual Meeting of the Radiological Society of North America. November 30,2005. Chicago III as quoted by Latchaw et al [3].
12. Ay H, Oliveira-Filho J, Buonanno FS. Et al. Diffusion-weighted imaging identifies a subset of lacunar infarction associated with embolic source. *Stroke* 1999;30:2644-2650 (abstract).
13. The National Institute Neurological Disorders and Stroke. rtPA Stroke study group. Tissue plasminogen activator for acute ischaemic stroke. *Engl J Med* 1995; 333:1581-87.
14. The European Cooperative Acute Stroke Study (ECASS). *JAMA* 1995; 274: 1017-1025.
15. Clark WM, Wissman S, Albers GW, Jhamandas JH, Madden P, Hamilton S. et al. Recombinant tissue-type plasminogen activator (Alteplase) for ischaemic stroke

3to 5 hours after symptom onset. The ATLANTIS Study: a randomzed controlled trial. Alteplase Thrombolysis for Acute Non-interventional Therapy in Ischaemic Stroke. *JAMA* 1999; 282: 2019-2026.

16. Zeevi N, Chhabra J, Silverman IE, Lee NS, McCullough LD. Acute stroke management in the elderly. *Cerebrovasc Dis* 2007; 25: 304-308.

17. Wardlow JM, Murray V, Berge E et al. Recombinant tissue plasminogen activator for ischaemic stroke: an updated systematic review and meta-analysis. *Lancet* 2012;379:2364-72.

18. Power M. An update on thrombolysis for acute ischaemic stroke. *ACNR* 2004; 4: 36-

19. Wahlgren N, Ahmed N, Davalos A, Ford GA, Grond M, Hacke W et al. Thrombolysis with alteplase for acute ischaemic stroke in the Safe Implementation of Thrombolysis in Stroke-Monitoring Study (SITS-MOST): an observational study. *Lancet* 2007; 369: 275-282.

20. Katzan L, Furlan AJ, Lloyd LE, Franl JI, Harper DL, Hinchey JA. et al. Use of tissue type plasminogen activator of acute ischaemic stroke. The Cleveland area experience. *JAMA* 2000; 263: 1151-58.

21. Flint AC, Duckwiler GR, Budzik RF, Liebeskind DS, Smith WS. Mechanical thrombectomy of intracranial internal carotid occlusion: pooled results of the MERCI and Multi MERCI Part 1 trials. *Stroke* 2007; 38(4): 1274-80.

22. Fiorella D, Levy EL, Turk AS, Albuquerque FC, Niemann DB, Aagaard-Kienitz B et al. US multicenter experience with te wingspan stent system for the treatment of intracranial atheromatous disease: periprocedural results. *Stroke*.2007; 38: 881-887.

23. Subramaniam S, Hilld MD. S. Decompressive hemicraniotomy for malignant middle cerebral artery infarction. *The Neurologist* 2009; 15: 178-184.

24. Hacke W, Schwab S, Horn M, Spranger M, De Georgia M, von Kummer R et al. Malignant middle cerebral artery territory infarction: clinical course and clinical signs. *Arch Neurol* 1996; 53: 309-315.

25. Schwab S, Steiner T, Aschoff A. et al. Early hemicraniectomy in patients with complete middle cerebral artery infarction. *Stroke* 1998;29:1888-1893.

26. Arac A, Blanchard V, Lee M, Steinberg G. Assessment of outcome following decompressive craniectomy for malignant middle cerebral artery infarction in patients older than 60 years. *Neurosurg Focus* 2009;26(6): E3 doi 10.3171/2009/3.FOCUS 0958 (abstract).

27. Schneck MJ. Hemicraniotomy for hemispheric infarction and HAMLET study:a sequel is needed. *The Lancet Neurology* 2009; 8(4): 303-304. [abstract].

28. Bhalla A, Wolfe CD, Rudd AG. Management of acute parameters after stroke QJM 2001; 94: 167-172.

29. Fuentes B, Ortegra-Cararrubios MA, San Jose B. Persistent hyperglycaemia >155mg/dl in acute ischaemic stroke patients. How well are we correcting it? Implications for outcome. Stroke 2010; 4: 2362-2365.

30. Oppenheimer SM, Hachinski VC. The cardiac consequences of stroke. *Neurol Clin* 1992; 10(1): 167-76.

31. Britton M, Carlsson A, de Faire U. Blood pressure course in patients with acute stroke and matched controls. *Stroke*;1986;17:861-4.

32. Sandser EC, Bath PM, Boysen G et al. The angiotensin-receptor blocker candesartan for treatment of acute stroke (CAST):a randomized, placebo-controlled, double-blind trial. *Lancet* 2011;377:741-50.

33. Jeffry I, Saver JL., Kalafut M. Thrombolysis therapy in stroke: Treatment and Medication. e-medicine http://emedicine.medscope.com/article/116080:treatments

34. Ronning OM, Guldvig B. Should stroke victims routinely receive supplemental oxygen? *Stroke* 1999;30:2053-2037.

35. Metawally Y. Cardiac consequences of stroke. http://yassermetwally.com

36. Oppenheimer SM. Neurogenic cardiac effects of cardiovascular disease. *Curr Opin in Neurol* 1994; 7(1):20-4.

37. Mayer SA. Recombinant activated Factor VII for acute intracerebral haemorrhage. *Stroke* 2007; 38: 763-767.

38. Wang DZ, Talkad AV. Treatment of intracerebral haemorrhage. What should we do now? *Curr Neurol Neurosci Rep.* 2009; 9 (11):13-18.

39. Mayer SA, Brun NC, Broderick J, Davis S, Dringer MN, Skelnick SE et al. Safety feasability of recombinant Factor VII for acute intracerebral haemorrhage. *Stroke* 2005b; 36: 74-79.

40. Barclay L, Vega C. American Heart and American Stroke Associations endorse New Stroke Guidelines. *http://cme.medscape.com/viewarticle/511995*

41. Adams HP Jr, Brott TG, Furlan AJ et al. Guidelines for thrombolytic therapy for acute stroke: a supplementto the guidelines for the mamnagement of acute ischaemic stroke: a statement for healthcare professionals from a special writing group of the Stroke Council, American Heart Association. *Circulation* 1996;94:1167-1174.

42. Broderick JP, Adams HP, Barson W, Feinberg W, Feldman E, Grotta J et al. Guidelines for the management of spontaneous intracerebral haemorrhage. *Stroke* 1999; 30: 905-912.

43. Amar AP. Controversies in the neurosurgical management of cerebellar haemorrhage and infarction. *Neurosurg* Focus 2012;32(4) EI doi 10.3171/2012.2 FOCUS 11369.

44. Dromerick A, Reding M. Medical and neurological complications during in patient stroke rehabilitation. *Stroke* 1994;25:358-361.

9

REHABILITATION OF

STROKE IN THE ELDERLY

The aim of rehabilitation in stroke survivors is to aid physical recovery, improve function, and enhance their quality of life. Number of studies have identified that age is an important prognostic factor for recovery following stroke[1]. It is believed that the elderly with stroke will have a poorer outcome compared to the younger stroke patients and the success rate of stroke rehabilitation is lower in the older patients[2]. The elderly stroke survivors with their multiple disabilities impair outcome and are more likely to need long—term care in aged—care facilities. Epidemiologic and demographic trends of populations particularly in developing countries suggest the burden of stroke is set to rise over the coming decades[3]. Stroke in the elderly will be in the near future a major health issue with significant cost implications as those who are disabled will require a variety of health care and assistance.

One of the strategies gaining popularity is the establishment of specialized stroke units for stroke rehabilitation. With the creation of specialized stroke rehabilitation units, the benefits of stroke units may be influenced by age and the problems associated with ageing[2]. The extra needs of the elderly are better met in the specialized units rather than in the general ward. Several studies have demonstrated the benefits of stroke unit rehabilitation regardless of age and the need for additional therapy in facilitating functional recovery[4,5,6,7]. There are often small variations between young and the elderly groups, that can be explained by age alone but this fact alone should not deny elderly stroke patients to rehabilitation based solely on advanced age[8].

Brain recovery may take place by several mechanisms. Neuroplasticity refers to the brain's ability to restructure itself and can take various forms. Collateral sprouting from intact cells to the dennervated region or unmasking of neural pathways and synapse formation not only in the spared regions of the damaged hemisphere but also in the sensorimotor cortex of the hemisphere contralateral to the injury[9,10]. Soon after a stroke there is initial improvement which last for a few weeks and is largely due to the resolution of associated local factors such as oedema, penumbra-ischaemic metabolic injury, diachisis[11], blood pressure among others. Another step in the recovery which begins early and can last for several months is neuroplasticity[11] which refers to the brain's ability to restructure itself following task specific repetitive exercises and workout, making restitution for loss function.

Stroke results in damage to the brain causing a number of deficits in the different neurological domains most commonly to the motor system. Other deficits include sensory disturbancs, problems of using or understanding language, cognition, memory and behaviour. Motor defects are the most common impairments after acute stroke and persist in nearly half of all patients[12]. Between one-third to two-thirds of stroke patients loose functional ability in their more affected arm and hand[13]. There are new options, therapy interventions and devices to help stroke patients to regain motor function. Matching specific impairments to different rehabilitation techniques, improvements in arm function were seen with constraint induced movement therapy (CIMT), electromyographic biofeedback and robotics[14]. i. Constraint—Induced Movement Therapy (CIMT):With loss of motor area's function the affected limb is not used and is compensated by the use of the normal limb. CIMT will be retraining the affected side and strengthening the good side to take over the weak side. It consists of the forced use of the affected limb by restricting the use of the non-affected limb by immobilizing the non-affected arm[15]. After damage to the motor cortex changes of activation have been observed in other motor areas. Constraint-Induced Movement Therapy (CIMT) an has shown great promise. ii. Robotic therapy: Robotic assisted therapy and automated computer programs are effective in reducing motor impairment. iii. Functional electrical stimulation (FES) has been shown to enhance motor recovery after stroke and can strengthen muscles, increase range of movements, reduce spastcity and prevent contractures.

Small lesions in the sensory motor cortex lead to changes in the excitatory and inhibitory neurotransmitter systems. Sensory impairments may occur in up to 60% of stroke patients[16]. There is very little rehabilitation research and studies on sensory interventions and sensory retraining after stroke. A systematic review supported passive and non active sensory training protocols[17].

There is growing evidence to indicate that visual rehabilitative strategies can reduce visual field defects and improve function[18]. Task specific and repetitive exercises appear to be key factors in promoting synaptogenesis and are core elements in rehabilitation following stroke[19] regardless of the impairment or technique[16]. Specific rehabilitation interventions for dysphagia and dysarthria include compensatory strategies and physical fitness training, high-intensity therapy and repetitive task training improved walking speed[16].

The management of complications both medical and neurological plays an important role in inpatient stroke rehabilitation[20]. Elderly patients have a high incidence of recurrent stroke together with co-morbidities and have a poorer outcome.

Spasticity, spasms, spastic dystonia

Spasticity is characterized by increased tone, exaggerated reflexes, clonus, and muscle spasms resulting from an upper motor neurone lesion. Injury to the motor system may be accompanied by spasticity, spastic dystonia, abnormal postures and findings such as weakness, fatigue, loss of dexterity and balance. The incidence varies from from 28-38% [21,22] to approximately 50% [12,23]. It can result in considerable pain, decreased function and in contracture. It is a leading cause of disability and long term disability. The degree of spasticity can vary in location and in severity from mild muscle stiffness to severe painful muscle spasms with abnormal postures a contractures. Although in some circumstances it may be beneficial usually it is injurious to the patient's function.

Whether spasticity associated with stroke need to be treated remains a subject of continuing investigation[24]. However spasticity and post—stroke shoulder pain should be treated[25]. Treatments include stretching, splinting, exercises or surgery for contracture. Consideration should be given to the use of medications such as dantrolene, oral baclofen, tizanidine or botulinum toxin. There is some data as to the usefulness of oral baclofen in stroke[26] but can cause significant sedation and have less impact on stroke-related spasticity[27]. Dantrolene however has restricted trial data to support its use in stroke but has no cognitive side effects[28]. Botulinum toxin injections have been recommended for selected patients with spasticity due to stroke[23,29].

Shoulder subluxation

Shoulder subluxation after stroke is characterized by partial or incomplete dislocation of the shoulder joint. The incidence varies from 17%[30] to approximately 81%[31]. It is a common problem with hemiplegia or weakness of musculature of the upper limbs[32]. There are several factors contributing to the occurrence some of which are related to the joint such as rotator cuff, reflex sympathetic dystrophy, inferior-anterior subluxation of the head of humerus and others related to the neurological lesion namely, spasticity, unilateral neglect, lack of sensibility ands central stroke pain[33]. Shoulder pain can impede rehabilitation and is associated with poorer outcomes and longer hospital stay[34].

The shoulder should be kept in the ideal position at all times and movements of the shoulder and upper limb carried out with the utmost care. Treatment entails the use of heat or ice packs, analgesics, support device and strapping of the shoulder(sling). Overhead pulleys should be avoided. Treatments include Functional electrical stimulation (FES) early after the onset of stroke[35] and intra-articular injections (triamcinalone) in patients with shoulder pain. Other treatments include hydrotherapy, acupuncture and muscle-toning with strengthening exercises and improving range of movements through stretching and mobilization techniques.

Shoulder Hand Syndrome (SHS)

SHS is characterized by pain and limitation of movement of the shoulder, wrist and hand with swelling followed by atrophy of the muscles and osteoporosis of the underlying bones. It is a form of reflex sympathetic dystrophy. The prevalence is rated at 12.5%—27% in stroke patients[36]. There are a number of factors involved in its etiology such as the severity of the stroke, recovery of motor deficit, spasticity, sensory disturbances together with subluxation of the shoulder joint[37]. It begins in the shoulder 1-6 months after stroke and develops in three stages. In the acute stage there is pain and tenderness with flushing, blanching and sweating and patchy bone thinning on X'ray. This is followed by the dystrophic stage with early skin changes, thickening of skin and contracture. There is persistent pain but swelling is reduced. In the atrophic stage there is reduced motion and function of the hand followed by contracture and thinning of the skin. The underlying bones on X'ray show osteoporosis. Treatment includes medications, physical therapy, psychotherapy, regional anaesthesia and sympathectomy[35].

Post-stroke dystonia

The term 'dystonia' refers to abnormal fluctuations in muscle tone produced by normal patterns of muscle contraction and phasic movements of various types such as tremors and dystonic spasms. Such abnormalities occur in a variety of neurological disorders and dystonia following hemiplegia is well recognized[38,39,40].

The anatomical basis of dystonia is not clear but radiographic data suggest the basal ganglia and in particular the putamen as the site[41]. It usually appears with improvement of the hemiplegia and is said to be due to an anberrant central nervous system sprouting consequent to a non-progressive cerebral insult[42]. Disruption of the thalamic output to the frontal cortex may produce dystonia resulting from the release of premotor control activity from thalamic control[37].

Post-stroke depression (PSD), emotionalism, anxiety

30% [43] to 40% [44] of stroke patients develop depression either in the early or late stages after stroke. It is the most common complication stroke survivors experience during inpatient stroke rehabilitation[45]. It is a common complication of stroke and a leading cause of increased mortality and morbidity and can impede rehabilitation process[46]. PSD is associated with a poor prognosis and may hinder recovery. SSRIs such as fluoxetine appear to improve recovery. Randomized controlled trials have demonstrated the efficacy of serataline, citalopram and nortripyline[44]. Although tricyclics and SSRIs appear effective the latter may be preferred in stroke because of their prompt action and better side effect profile[45]. The elderly with depression hospitalized for geriatric rehabilitation are at high risk of falls associated with use of anti-depressants must be borne in mind in the context of their potential benefit[46].

Apart from depression there a a variety of neuropsychiatric sequelae seen after stroke[47]. It is not uncommon to see post stroke patients exhibiting emotionalism and about 15% of them show extreme form of emotional change—' uncontrollable laughter/crying and if not treated develop clinical depression[47]. Another psychiatric syndrome is anxiety and co-exists with post stroke depression and is often undiagnosed[48]. General Anxiety Disorder accompanying post stroke depression delays recovery from depression and reduces overall social functioning[49].

Post-stroke fatigue

Post-stroke fatigue (PSF) is a common sequel to stroke but often is underdiagnosed. It is important to recognize PSF for it can impede recovery and rehabilitation[50] and may have a negative impact on the quality of life and daily functioning[51]. Sleep disorders, sleep disordered breathing, limited exercise capacity and increased gait energy cost can be related to physical fatigue [52]. It occurs in 30-72% of stroke survivors[52,53,54] but few studies have documented its high frequency[50]. Little is known of the pathogenesis. The causes are multifactorial and besides stroke it can be associated with other disorders such as multiple sclerosis, Human immunodeficiency Virus, AIDs and cancer. There is an association with brain stem and thalamic lesions in stroke. Staub and Bogousslasky[50]postulated a concept that 'primary' post-stroke fatigue may be linked to attentional deficits resulting from specific damage to the reticular formation and related structures involved in subcortical attentional network. Table 9.1 summarises the different characteristics of some post-stroke complications.

Table 9.1 summarises the different characteristics in some post-stroke complications

Syndrome	Spasticity, spasms, dystonia	Shoulder subluxation	Shoulder hand syndrome	Post-stroke depression Emotional-ism anxiety	Post-stroke fatigue
Frequency	28-38% [21,22]	17-81% [30,31]	12-27% [36]	30-40% [43,44]	30-72% [52,53,54]
Patho-genesis	UMN lesion	hemiplegia, weakness of upper limb muscle, rotator cuff	stroke severity spasticity subluxation with sensory disturbances reflex sympathetic dystrophy	structural changes in frontal, subcortical, medial temporal	multifactorial ?brain stem and thalamic lesioons
Clinical	pain, loss of dexterity, reduced function	pain	pain, tenderness sweating, flushing dystrophy, atrophy	Psychomot-or retardation	physical fatigue

Treatment	stretching, splinting, medication	ice-packs strapping, sling FES, intra-articular injections hydrotherapy acupuncture	medications, physical, regional anaesthesia, sympathectomy[36]	SSRIs tricyclics [44]	
Sequelae	contracture abnormal postures	impede rehabilitation, poor outcome	reduced function contracture, osteoporosis	leading cause of mortality & morbidity, high risk of fall	impede recovery, daily functioning & QOL [49,50]

The sequence of recovery is shown in Table 9.2. There are several impediments such as depression, poor motivation, severe motor deficit, perceptual impairment, poor pre stroke health, communication disabilities and impaired cognition, factors which may retard recovery. Post-stroke recovery shows differing patterns across varied areas of neurological function. For example in 95% of the patients maximum arm motor function is achieved by 9 weeks[55] and in 95% of patients formal level of language function by 6 weeks [26].

Table 9.2 Sequence of recovery

Level of counciousness improves

Head and neck control with improved balance sitting up

Truncal control with balance on standing

Limb control proximal to distal flaccidity to spasticity

Functional recovery

PREVENTION of recurrent stroke

The acute hospitalization is focused not only on treatment of the acute stroke but also in identifying risk factors for recurrent stroke. Poststroke outpatient care is largely rehabilitation and prevention of recurrent stroke. The risk factors for stroke include hypertension, diabetes, hyperlipidaemia, diabetes and life style factors such as smoking, alcohol abuse, diet and activity (see Chapter 13).

* The aim of stroke rehabilitation is to help the stroke survivor to return to meaningful roles in life.
* The extra needs of the elderly are better met in the specialized units rather than in the general ward.
* Although there are variations beteween young and the elderly, the elderly stroke patients should not be denied rehabilitation based solely on advanced age.
* Neuroplasticity refers to the brain's ability to restructure itself.
* There are now new options, therapy, interventions and devices to help stroke patients to regain motor function.
* Rehabilitation techniques include Constraint-Induced Movement Therapy (CMT), Robotic therapy and Functional electrical stimulation (FES) among others.
* The management of complications both medical and neurological plays an important role in inpatient stroke rehabilitation.
* Some of the complications post-stroke seen in the rehabilitation unit include spasticity, spastic dystonia, spasms, shoulder subluxation, shoulder hand syndrome, post-stroke depression, emotionalism, anxiety and post-stroke fatigue.
* There are several barriers to recovery such as depression, poor motivation, severe motor deficit, perceptual impairment, impaired cognition, poor pre stroke health and communication disabilities.
* After discharge from hospital the basic issues are secondary prevention strategies and patient adherence to post-stroke rehabilitation guidelines.

REFERENCES

1. Jongbloed L. Prediction of function after stroke. A critical review. *Stroke* 1986;17:383, 389.
2. Kalra L. Does age affect benefits of stroke unit rehabilitation? *Stroke*; 1994;25:346, 351.
3. Young J, Forster A. Review of stroke rehabilitation. *BMJ* 2007; 334: 86-90.
4. Kalra L, Dale P, Crome P. Improving stroke rehabilitation: a controlled study. *Stroke* 1993; 24: 1462-1467.
5. Friedman PJ. Stroke rehabilitation in the elderly: a new patient management system. *NZ Med J* 1990; 103: 234-236.
6. Indredavik B, Bakke F, Solberg R et al. Benefit of stroke unit: a randomized controlled trial. *Stroke* 1991; 22: 1026-1031,
7. Garraway WM, Ambler AJ, Prescott RJ, Hockey L. Management of acute stroke in the elderly:preliminary results of a controlled trial. *BMJ* 1980; 280: 1040-1043.
8. Bagg S, Pombo AO, Hopman W. Effect of age on functional outcomes after stroke rehabilitation. *Stroke* 2002;33:179-185.
9. Kozlowski DA, Schaller T. Relationship between dendritic pruning and behaviour recovery following sensorimotor cortex lesions. *Behav Brain Res* 1998; 97: 89-98.
10. Stroemer RP, Kent TA, Hulsebosch CE. Neocortical neural sprouting, synaptogenesis, and behavioural recovery after neocortical infarction in rats. *Stroke* 1995; 26: 2135-2144.
11. Teasell R, McClure A. B. The Principles of Stroke Rehabilitation. http:www. ebrsr.com/-ebrsr/uploads/B_Principles_of_Stroke_Rehabilitation_(Full_Version).pdf. accessed 15 2.2013.
12. Rathore SS, Hinn AR, Cooper LS et al. Characterization of incidence stroke signs and symptoms: findings from the Atherosclrosis Risk in Communities Study. *Stroke* 2002; 33: 27 18-2721.
13. Fritz SL, Light KE, Patterson TS. et al. Active finger extension predicts outcomes after constraint-induced movement therapy for individuals with hemiparesis after stroke. *Stroke* 2005; 36: 1172-1177.
14. Langhorne P, Coupar F, Pollock A. Motor recovery after stroke: a systematic review *Lancet Neurol* 2009; 8:741-754.
15. Liepert J, Miltner WHR, Bauder H et al. Motor cortex plasticity during constraint-induced movement therapy in stroke patients. *Neurosci Lett.* 1998; 250: 5-8
16. Kalra L. Stroke Rehabiliation 2009. Old Chestnuts and New Insights. *Stroke* 2010; 41: e88-e90.
17. SM, Hillier S. Evidence for there training of sensation after stroke: a systematic review. *Clin Rehabil* 2009; 23: 27-39.

18. Plow EB, Maguire S, Obretenova S. et al. Approaches to rehabilitation for visual field defects following brain lesions. *Expert Rev Med Devices* 2009; 6: 291-305.

19. O'Dell M et al. Stroke rehabilitation-Strategies to enhance motor recovery. *Ann Rev Med*. Feb 2009.

20. Dobkin B. Neuromedical complications in stroke patients transferred for rehabilitation before and after diagnostic related groups. *J Neuro Rehabil* 1987; 1:3-7.

21. Sommerfield DK, Elsy U-B Eck PT, Svensson A-K et al. Spasticity after stroke: its occurrence and association with motor impairments and activity limitation. *Stroke* 2004; 35: 134-140

22. Watkins CL, Leathley MJ, Gregson JM et al. Prevalence of spasticity post stroke. *Clin Rehab* 2002; 16(5): 515-522.

23. Gresham GE, Duncan PW, Stason KB et al. Post stroke rehabilitation Clinical Practice Guidelines. No 16. Rockville, Md: US Department of Health and Human Services, Public Health Services, Aging for Health Care Policy and Research May 1995. AHCPR Publication No. 95-0662.

24. Cramer SC. Editorial Comment-Spasticity after stroke: What's the catch. *Stroke* 2004; 35: 131-140.

25. Barclay L, Vega C. Amerivcan Heart and American Stroke Associations endorse New Stroke Guidelines. Website: http://cme.medscape.com/viewarticle/511995.

26. Milanod IG. Mechanisms of baclofen action in spasticity. *Acta Neurol Scand* 1991; 85: 305-310

27. Pedersen E, Arlein-Soborog P, Mai J. The mode of action of the gaba derivative baclofen in human spasticity. *ActaNeurol Scand* 1974; 50: 665-85.

28. Ketel WB, Kolb ME. Long term treatment with dantrolene sodium of stroke patients with spastiity limiting the return of function. *Curr Med Res Opin* 1984; 9:161-169.

29. Royal College of Physicians Clinical Guidelines for Stroke 2nd ed. Prepared by Intercollegiate Stroke Working Parthy. London RCP, 2004.

30. Fitzgerald-Finch OP, Gibson JM. Subluxation of the shoulder in hemiplegia. *Age Aging* 1975; 4: 16-18.

31. Najenson T, Pikielny SS. Malalignment of the glenohumeral joint following hemiplegia. *Amer Phys Med* 1965; 8:96-99.

32. Seneviratne C, Then KL, Reimer M. Post stroke shoulder subluxation: a concern for neurosciences nurses. *Axone* 2005; 27(1): 26-31.

33. H, Chantraine L. Shoulder pain in hemiplegia revisited: contribution of functional electrical stimulation and other therapies. *J Rehabil Med* 2003; 35: 49-54.

34. Turner-Stokes L, Jackson D. Shoulder pain after stroke: a review of the evidence base to inform the development of an integrated care pathay. *Clin Rehab* 2002; 16(3): 276-298.

35. Vuagnat H, Chantraine A. Shoulder pain in hemiplegia revisited: contribution of functional electrical stimulation and other therapies. J Rehabil Med 2003; 35(2):49-54 (abstract).

36. Zyluk X, Zyluk B. Shoulder hand syndrome in patients after stroke. *Neuro Neurochir Pol* 1999; 33(1): 131-142. in Polish (abstract).

37. Pertoldi S, Benedetto P. Shoulder hand syndrome after stroke: A complex regional pain syndrome. *Eura Med. cophjs.* 2005; 41: 283-292.

38. Marsden CD, Obeso JA, Zarrang JJ et al. The anatomical basis of symptomatic dystonia. *Brain* 1985;108: 463-483.

39. Grimes JD, Hassan MN, Quarrington AM, A'Alton J. Delayed onset of post-hemiplegic dystonia: demonstration of basal ganglia pathology. *Neurology* 1982; 32: 1033-5.

40. Nagaratnam N. Letter to editor. Post-hemiplegic dystonia allowing right anterior cerebral artery infarction. *Aust NJ 1991*; 21: 381-382.

41. Koller WC. Letter to editor. *Neurology* 1985; 35: 615.

42. Burke RE, Fahn S, Gold AP. Delayed onset dystonia in patient with static encephalopathy. *J Neurol Neurosurg Psych.* 1980; 73: 789-97.

43. Paolucci S. Epidemiology and treatment of post stroke depression. *Neuropsychiatr Dis Treat* 2008; 4(1): 145-54.

44. Starkstein SE, Mizrahi R, Power BD. *Expert Opin Pharmacother* 2008; 9(8): 291-8.

45. Turner-Stokes L, Hassan N. Depression after stroke: a review of the evidence base to inform the development of an integrated care pathway. Part 2. Treatment alternatives. *Clin Rehab* 2002; 16(3): 248-60.

46. Aizen E, Shugaev I, Lenger R. Risk factors and characteristics of falls during inpatient rehabilitation of elderly patients. *Arch Geront Geriatrics* 2007; 44: 1-12.

47. Robinson RG. The Clinical Neuropsychiatry of stroke. New York. Cambridge University Press,1998.

48. Castillo CS, Robinson RG. Focal neuropsychiatric syndromes after cerebrovascular disease. *Curr Opin Psychiatry* 1993; 6: 109112.

49. Shimada K, Robinson RG. Effects of anxiety disorder on impairment and recovering from stroke. *J Neuropsychiatry Clin Neuro Sci* 1998; 10: 34-40.

50. Staub F, Bogousslavsky J. Fatigue after stroke: a major but neglected issue. *Cerebrovasc Dis* 2001; 12(2): 75-81.

51. De Groot MH, Phillips ST, Eskes GA. Fatigue associated with stroke and other associated conditions: implications for stroke rehabilitation. *Arch Phys Med Rehabil* 2003; 84(10):1714-20.

52. Colle F, Bonan I, Gilliz LMC et al. Fatigue after stroke. *Ann Readapt Med Phys* 2006; 48(6): 272-6.

53. Pak JY, Chun MH, Kang SH et al. Functional outcome in post-stroke patients with and without fatigue. *Am J Phys Med Rehabil* 2009;88(7): 554-8.

54. Jaracz K, Mielcarek L, Kozubski W. Clinical and psychological correlations of post-stroke fatigue. Preliminary results. *Neuro Neurochir Pol.* 2007; 41(1): 34-43.

55. Nakayama H, Jorgensen H, Raaschou H, Olsen T. Recovery of upper extremity function in stroke patients: the Copenhagen Stroke Study. *Arch Phys Med Rehabil* 1994;75: 394-398.

10

TRANSIENT ISCHAEMIC ATTACK (TIA)

A transient ischaemic attack (TIA) is a circulatory event which produces a focal neurological deficit with complete recovery within 24 hours. With the advent of sophisticated neuroimaging techniques the definition of TIA has unfolded to less than one hour episode of focal dysfunction with no imaging evidence of acute infarction. The American Heart Association and American Stroke Association (AHA/ASA) 2009 Guidelines endorsed this new definition but omitted the phrase, 'less than one hour'[1].

Magnetic resonance imaging (MRI) especially diffusion-weighted magnetic resonance has demonstrated that in one—third of the patients with proven TIA have ischaemic changes. These patients with MRI changes have a different clinical course compared to those without MRI changes[2,3]. Imaging was found to be important in assessing stroke recurrence risk. It was shown that CT or MRI findings of present or recent infarcts were found to correlate with higher early risks[4,5]. However this factor mainly applies to TIA patients[6]. Nonetheless, irrespective of the definition, TIA remains within the spectrum of ischaemic events with a notable increase in risk of stroke. There is considerable evidence that the risk of stroke is more than 10% in the 90 days after TIA[7,8,9].

Incidence prevalence and epidemiology

An estimated 32,000 Australians suffer a first ever stroke each year[10] and a similar number are affected by TIA[11]. The overall prevalence of TIA is 7% in males and 4.9% in females. This increased with age reaching 10.2% in males and 7.4% in females and decreased in subjects of both sexes aged 85 years or over[12]. TIA was substantially higher among blacks and women than among whites and men. Those with TIA and hypertension experienced higher stroke incidence rates and 13% of those with TIA had evidence of cardiovascular disease[13]. Three populations were studied in Central Spain with regards to prevalence rate of cerebrovascular disease, stroke and TIA. Age-specific prevalence rates of all three increased exponentially with advancing age and was higher in men than for women. The prevalence rates were also higher in the suburban area[14]. A Korean study reported that in a random sampled 714 community dwelling Koreans aged >65 years the prevalence of stroke and TIA were higher in Korean elders than in white elders[15].

Pathophysiology

About 40% of patients with ischaemic stroke syndromes have extracranial arterial lesions accessible to surgery[16] most commonly carotid stenosis[17]. An estimated 80,000 Australians between the ages 50-74 years have significant carotid stenosis[18]. The most common cause is an embolus from the atherosclerotic plaque in one of the cartotid arteries or from a thrombus in the heart. Large vessel disease (especially high grade carotid stenosis) and cardioembolism (atrial fibrillation and severely diseased and replaced valves) carry higher risks of stroke recurrence[6]. In the former the stroke risk was found to be 12.6% within 1month and 19.2% at 3 months and in the latter it was estimated to be 4.6% within a month[19].

Symptomatology

The symptoms of TIA vary widely depending on the area of brain involved. The presentation of TIA symptoms can often be divided according to the vascular territories involved, anterior (carotid) circulation and posterior (vertebrobasilar) circulation. It is important to distinguish between them if carotid endarterectomy is to be considered although the clinical distinction can be difficult. Despite this there are clinical features that are more likely to be allied to one or the other.

Anterior circulation TIA (carotid TIAs):Transient occlusion of the ophthalmic artery will result in monocular blindness (TMB) or amaurosis fugax and described by the patient as a 'curtain' descending over the affected eye. It may also manifest as a transient hemispheric episode (Table 10.1).

Posterior circulation TIA: Any one of these symptoms shown in Table 10.1 may be an isolated symptom of posterior circulation involvement but for isolated vertigo without other symptoms is most unlikely to be caused by vertebrobasilar disease.

Table 10.1. Anterior circulation and
Posterior circulation TIAs

monocular blindness	diplopia
unilateral weakness	dysarthria
unilateral numbness	ataxia
clumsiness of hand	vertigo
dysphasia	blurred vision
dysarthria	transient global amnesia

Differential diagnosis

There are many non-vascular conditions that may cause symptoms suggestive of TIA or stroke and have often been referred to as 'TIA mimics' or 'stroke mimics'[20] The most common mimics are hypoglycaemia, migraine, seizures, post-ictal states and tumours. Hypoglycaemia manifests with confusion, visual disturbances, inappropriate behaviour and accompanied by sweating, tremulousness, hunger and diminished level of consciousness or coma[21]. Transient hypoglycaemia may simulate a stroke like event with hemiplegia and aphasia[22]. Hypoglycaemia can be excluded by appropriately timed blood sugar levels.

Migraine occurs in young and middle-aged patients and is characterised by headache often unilateral and an aura which precedes the headache. If the patient has not had migraine headaches in the past, this diagnosis should not be made until all other possibilities are excluded[23]. In syncopal attack there is transient loss of consciousness and loss of postural tone, a feeling of uneasiness and fear which may indicate impending loss of consciousness. However, cardiac—related syncope typically begins and ends abruptly.

Todd's paralysis is characterized by temporary usually unilateral weakness and may last for 36-48 hours following a seizure. Partial epileptic seizures are accompanied by convulsive movements of the limbs and takes a few seconds to few minutes for the symptoms to start then involves other areas. There have been reports of stroke and TIA symptoms with chronic subdural haematoma[24]. Transient global amnesia appears suddenly with confusion, disorientation and lasts as long as 2 hours or more together with retrograde memory deficit[23].

In Transient Monocular Blindnes (TMB) or Amaurosis Fugax the visual disturbance or loss such as blindness, dimming or blurring affects one eye for seconds or minutes[25]. It may occur alone or in combination with TIA. Differential diagnosis of TMB includes ocular events such as vitreous detachment, central retinal vein thrombosis, intraocular haemorrhage, intermittent angle chronic glaucoma, and vasospasm/angiospasm[26].

Diagnosis and evaluation of a patient with suspected TIA

Medical history of specific symptoms and thorough neurological and cardiovascular examinations provide the most important information to diagnose a TIA. TIA poses considerable difficulty in diagnosis and diagnostic uncertainity is common. A third of patients referred to a TIA/stroke clinic have a non-vascular cause[29] and only 22% of primary care physicians knew of the definition of TIA[30]. The Oxfordshire Community Stroke Study Project (OCSP) revealed, of the 512 patients referred by the General Practitioners or attending doctors with a possible diagnosis of TIA, 317 (62%) were considered not to have TIA by the study group neurologists[11].

Risk stratification

Patients presenting with TIA or minor stroke are at high risk of early stroke upto 10% in the first 48 hours[31]. The overall risk of stroke in patients with TIA has been found to be 8% within a week [9]and 20% with a 3-month period[32,33]. There are several scoring systems based on the clinical profile of patients used to determine the risk of early stroke recurrence after a TIA. Presently a validated score—the ABCD2 score is from 5 factors with 7 points[7]. The risk of stroke within 2 days following TIA with a score between 0-3 is 1%, 4-5 is 4.1% and 6-7 is 8.1% respectively[7]. Although validated in several studies the ABCD2 score is not wholly dependable in predicting carotid artery stenosis[34]. The ABCD2 score may act as a guide but what is important is the identification as to the mechanism and pathology of the TIA for these are what determine the risk of stroke and the treatment[35].

The predictive scores do not incorporate imaging findings which have been shown to have predictive value. CT results can improve prediction[36]. In spite of the transient nature of the symptoms diffusion-weighted imaging (DWI) has identified areas of acute brain ischaemia in about half the patients and with symptoms such motor impairment. The presence of ischaemic lesions on DWI correlates with several clinical features known to predict stroke risk such as dysarthria, dysphagia and motor weakness[37]. Clinical scores were not associated with a positive DWI [38]. Ipsilateral carotid stenosis (> or- 50%) and atrial fibrillation were associated with positive DWI [37]. The presence of multiple DWI lesions of varying ages suggests active early recurrence over time and portends a higher early risk of future ischaemic events[39]. In addition to ABCD2 score taking DWI into account improves the prediction of early risk of stroke after TIA[40]. The results suggest DWI evaluation should be done urgently after TIA[41] and the National Stroke Association guidelines suggest including imaging at some point [42].

Current international guidelines have adopted the ABCD2 score in risk stratification of patients with TIA[43]. Two large population studies investigating the diagnostic utility of ABCD2 for prediction of early risk after TIA and to evaluate whether carotid stenosis or atrial fibrillation might add to the prognostic yield of ABCD2 score noted that the degree of carotid stenosis was linearly associated with increased stroke risk after TIA whereas atrial fibrillation was not[44,45]. This highlights the importance of carotid evaluation in all TIA patients independent of the presenting ABCD2 scores[43].

Management

For a new onset TIA patient an ABCD2 can be a guide in the management and patients with a score of 4 or more crescendo TIA, atrial fibrillation and those on anticoagulants should be referred to the hospital for prompt evaluation and treatment[46]. The EXPRESS Study[47]demonstrated that intense and immediate medical treatment of TIA reduced the early risk of stroke by 80%. There is still however no consensus on the urgent treatment of TIA. Many advocate urgent presentation to hospital of all patients with evolving or resolved symptoms of TIA. According to the American Heart Association Guidelines a new onset TIA patient with an ABCD2 score of 3 or higher should be referred to the hospital immediately for emergent diagnostic evaluation[1] (Fig. 10.1). Low risk patients ABCD2 score below 3 can be managed by a specialist or referred to a neurological/TIA clinic and be seen within 7-10 days.

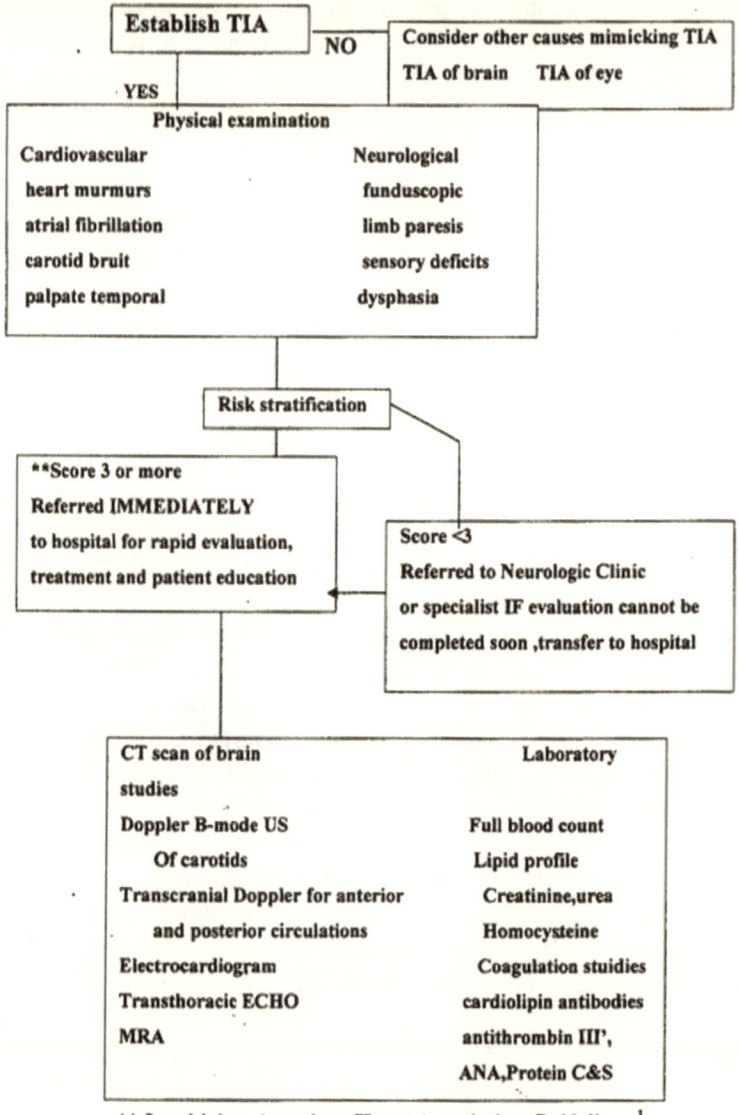

Fig.10.1. Algorithm in suspected Transient Ischaemic Attack

The mainstay of management of TIA following acute recovery is diagnosis and treatment of the underlying cause. The family physicians are advised to give aspirin at the time of diagnosis. CT scan must be done to exclude haemorrhage before commencement of antithrombotic therapy. Specialist assessment confers the diagnosis usually with cerebral imaging (prefereably with MRI) and carotid ultrasound to detect patients suitable for carotid endarterectomy[48.] Table 10.2 summarises the treatment and prevention of stroke in TIA patients. The American Heart Association (AHA) and the American Stroke Association(ASA) and the more recent guidelines from the 8th American College of Chest Physicians Conference on Antithrombotic and Antipalatelet therapy recommend asprin, clopidogrel or extended-release dipyramidole (ER-DP) plus aspirin as accepted first line options for secondary prevention of ischaemic events in patients with a history of TIA or stroke[49]. For patients with noncardioembolic TIA antiplatelet agents rather than oral anticoagulation are recommended to reduce cardiovascular events or recurrent stroke The recommended dose is Asprin (50 to 325 mg/d) monotherapy or combination of aspirin and extended—release dipyramidole and clopidegrol monotherapy according to the AHA/ASA recommendations[50].

The ESPS-2 trial demonstrated that aspirin 25 mg twice daily and dipyramidole in a modified release form at a dose of 200mg twice daily have each been equally effective for the secondary prevention of stroke and TIA[51]. When coprescribed the protective effects are additive. The combination being more significantly effective than either agent prescribed singly [51;52]. Low dose aspirin does not eliminate the propensity for induced bleeding[51] and in patients who are aspirin intolerant clopidogrel is another option but is said to have less advantage over aspirin than aspirin plus ER-DP and its combination with aspirin has only marginally better efficacy and increased bleeding risks[53].

Table 10.2. Treatment and prevention of stroke in TIA patients

	Mode of action	Dosage	Adverse	Efficacy	Comment
I. Antiplatelet therapy					
i. Aspirin	inhibits production of thromboxane	50-325mg daily	bleeding GI effects	reduced risk of stroke by 77%	cheap, safe
ii. Clopidogrel	inhibits platelet aggregration	75mg daily	bleeding neutropenia diarrhoea TTP*	9% reduction for ischaemic events	Alternative to aspirin
iii. Dipyridamole	disrupts platelet functions by inhibiting phosphodiesterase activity	100mg 6 hrly	headache dizziness GI upsets	reduces by 15% of stroke—death	
iv. Combination dipyridamole+ aspirin	see i and iii	200mg dipyridamole bd bd		23% reduction in TIA & stroke	option for patients on antiplatelet and stroke

127

v. Ticlopidine	inhibits platelets disrupting ADP pathway	500mg daily	TTP, * neutropenia	12% reduction compared to aspirin	risks > modest benefits
II. Anticoagulant therapy					
Warfarin	inhibits Vitami K	INR 2.5	bleeding	In AF reduces risk of stroke by 68%	to patients with cardio—embolic sources
III. Carotid Endarterectomy					
Recent TIA	severe stenosis (70-99%)			reduces risk of stroke by 48%	
Recent TIA	moderate stenosis (>50-69%)			reduces risk of stroke by about 27%	

*TIP. Thombotic thrombocytopenic purpura

Information sources: Adams et al,[50], Diener et al[51], Chaturvedi [52], Kirshner [53], Cina et al,[54]

* Irrespective of the definition, TIA remains within the spectrum of ischaemic events with a notable increase in risk of stroke.
* TIA is a medical emergency for it is not possible to predict if it will advance to a major stroke.
* The stroke rate is more than 10% in the 90 days of TIA and the patient with TIA has to be evaluated promptly as there is an increased risk of stroke.
* The most common cause is an embolus from the atherosclerotic plaque in one of the carotid arteries or from a thrombus in the heart.
* TIA mimics include hypoglycaemia, migraine, seizures, post-ictal state, tumours among others.
* Intense and immediate medical treatment of TIA reduces the early risk of stroke by 80% [47].
* The use of ABCD2 scoring scale to identify high and low risk TIA patients is confirmed but is important is the identification of the mechanisms and pathology of TIA.
* Carotid evaluation in all TIA patients is important and independent of the presenting ABCD2 scores.
* For non-cardioembolic TIA—antiplatelets agents are recommended. Aspirin (50-325mg/d) monotherapy or combination of aspirin and extended release dipyramidole and clopidergrol monotherapy[50].
* The combination being more significantly effective than either agent prescribed singly.

REFERENCES

1. Easton JD, Saver JL, Albers GW et al. Definition and evaluation of transient ischaemic attack: a scientific statement for health care professionals from the American Heart Association/American Stroke Association Council on Cardiovacular Radiology and Intervention, Council of cardiovascular Nursing and Interdisciplinary Council of Peripheral Vascular Disease. The American Academy of Neurology affirms the value of this statement as an educational tool for neurologists. *Stroke* 2009;40:2276-2293.

2. Ay H, Walker JK, Benner T et al. Transient ischaemic attack: a unique syndrome? *Ann Neurol* 2005; 57: 679-686.

3. Coutts S, Simon J, Elearzin M et al. Triaging transient ischaemic attack and minor stroke patients using acute magnetic resonance imaging. *Ann Neurol* 2005; 57: 848-854.

4. Douglas C, Johnston CM, Elkins J et al. Head computed tomography findings predict short-term stroke risk after transient ischaemic attack. *Stroke* 2003; 34: 2894-2899.

5. Purroy F, Montaner J, Rovira A et al. Higher risk of further vascular events among transient ischaemic attack patients with diffuse-weighted imaging acute ischaemic lesions. *Stroke* 2004; 35: 2313-2319.

6. Streifler JY. Early stroke risk after a transient ischaemic attack Can it be minimized? Editorial. *Stroke* 2008; 39: 1655-1656.

7. Johnston SC, Gress DR, Browner WS, Sidney S. Short-term prognosis after emergency-department diagnosis of transient ischaemic attack. *JAMA* 2000; 284: 2901-2906.

8. Eliassziw M, Kennedy J, Hill MD, et al. Early risk of stroke after a transient ischaemic attack in patients with internal carotid artery disese. *CMAJ* 2004; 170: 1105-1109.

9. Coull A, Lovett JK, Rothwell PM. On behalf of the Oxford Vascular Study. Population-based study of early risk of stroke after transient ischaemia attack or minor stroke: implications for public education and organization of services. *BMJ* 2004; 328: 326-328.

10. Anderson CS, Jameozck KD, Burvill PB et al. Ascertaining the true incidence of stroke: experience from the Perth Community Stroke Study. 1989-1990. *Med J Aust* 1993; 188: 80-84.

11. Dennis MS, Bamford J, Sandercock PHG, Warlow CP. Incidence of TIA in the Oxfordshire England. *Stroke* 1989; 20: 333-339.

12. Orlandi G, Gelli A, Fanucchi S. Prevalence of stroke and TIA in the elderly population of an Italian rural community. *Eur J Epidem* 2003; 18: 879-882 (abstract).

13. Ostfield AM, Shekella RB, Klawans HL. TIA a risk of stroke in elderly poor population. *Stroke* 1973; 4: 980 (abstract).

14. Diaz-Guzman J, Bermegon-Pariya F, Benito-Leon J et al. Prevalence of stroke and TIA in three elderly populations of Central Spain. *Neuroepidemiology* 2008; 30: 247-253.

15. Han MK, Hah Y, Lie SB et al. Prevalence of stroke and TIA in Korean elders. Findings from the Korean longitudinal study on health and ageing (LLoSHA). *Stroke* 2009; 40: 966-969.

16. Robun M, Baumit M. The national survey of stroke 1981; 12 (2Pc 2 Suppl1) 145-157.

17. Lord RSA. Short-stay carotid endarterectomy. Editorial *MJA* 1998; 168: 149-150.

18. National Health and Medical Research Council. Clinical practitioner guidelines: prevention of stroke. Canberra: *NHMRC* 1996.

19. Lovett JK, Coull AJ, Rothwell PM. Early risk of recurrence by subtype of ischaemic stroke in population—based incidence studies. *Neurology* 2004; 62: 569-573.

20. Pendlebury ST, Giles MF, Rothwell PM. Transient Ischaemic Attack and Stroke. Cambridge University Press. accessed website: *http://www.Cambridge. org/catalogue/catalogue.asp?isbn=9780521735124 &ss =exc* (accessed on 9/02/2010.

21. Malouf R, Brust JC. Hypoglycaemia causing neurological manifestations and outcome. *Ann Neurol* 1985;17:421-430

22. Montgomery BM, Pinner CA, Newberry SC. Transient hypoglycaemic hemiplegia. *Arch Int Med* 1964;114:680-684.

23. Hankey GJ. Stroke. Churchill Livingstone 2002.

24. Moster ML, Johnson DE, Reinmuth OM. Chronic subdural haematoma with transient neurological deficits: a review of 15 cases. *Ann Neurol* 1983;14:539-542.

25. Lord RS. Tansient monocular blindness. *Aust NZJ Ophthalmol* 1990;18:299-305.

26. Heckman JG, Garel C, Neundorfer B et al. Vasospastic Amaurosis fugax. *J Neutrol Neuosurg & Psychiatry*. 2003;24(2):149.

27. Mattsson P, Lundberg PO. Characteristics and prevalence of transient visual disturbances indicative of migraine visual aura. *Cephalagia* 1999;19(5):477-8

28. Cologino D, Torelli P, Manzoni GC. Transient visual disturbances during migraine without aural attacks. *Headache* 2002;42 (9): 930-3.

29. Martin DJ, Young G, Enevoldson TD, Hinfurey P. Over diagnosis of transient ischaemic attack and minor stroke: experience at a regional neurovascular clinic. *QJM* 1997; 90: 759-67.

30. Hogan N, Boenau I. The Emergent patient:Transient ischaemic attack. *Emerg Med*. 2006; 30(3): 41-46.

31. Rothwell P, Buchan A, Johnston S. Recent advances in management of transient ischaemic attacks and minor ischaemic strokes. *Lancet Neurol* 2005; 5: 33-331.

32. Kleindorfer D; Panagos P, Pancioli A et al. Incidence and short-term prognosis of transient ischaemic attack in a population-based study. *Stroke* 2005; 36: 720-724.

33. Johnston SC, Rothwell PM, Nguyen-Huyah MN et al. Validation and refinement of scores to predict very early stroke risk. after transient ischaemic attack. *Lancet* 2007; 269: 283-292.

34. Sivakumar R, Shinh N, Kingsworth B et al. Can we predict carotid stenosis by ABCD2 score or other clinical features? *Cerebrovasc Dis* 2008; 28 (suppl2) 171.

35. Blacker DJ. There's more to transient ischaemic attack than ABCD. *Int Med J* 2009; 39: 332-334.

36. Sciolla R, Melis F. Rapid identification of high-risk transient ischaemic attack. Prospective validation of the ABCD score. *Stroke* 2008; 39: 297-302.

37. Redgrave JN, Coutt SB, Schulz UG et al. Systematic review of associations between the presence of acute ischaemic lesions on diffusion-weighted imaging and clinical predictors of early stroke risk after transient ischaemic attack. *Stroke* 2007; 38(5): 1482-8.

38. Purroy F, Begue R, Quillez A et al. The California ABCD and unified ABCD2 rrisk scores and the presence of acute ischaemic lesions on diffusion-weighted imaging in TIA patients. *Stroke* 2009; 40(6): 2229-32.

39. Sylasja PN, Coults SB, Subramaniam S et al. Acute ischaemic lesions of varying ages predict risk of ischaemic events in stroke/TIA patients. *Neurology* 2007; 68(6): 415-9.

40. Calvet D, Touze E, Oppenheim C et al. DWI lesions and TIA etiology improve the prediction of stroke after TIA. *Stroke* 2009; 40(1): 187-92.

41. Sorenson AG. Advances in Imaging 2007. *Stroke* 2008; 39: 276-278.

42. Johnston SC, Nguyen-Huyeh, Schwarz ME et al. National Stroke Association guidelines for management of transient ishaemic attack. *Ann Neurol* 2006; 60: 301-304.

43. Tsivgoulis G, Heliopoulos J. Potential and failure of the ABCD2 score in stroke risk prediction after transient ischaemic attack. *Stroke* 2010; 41: 836-838.

44. Sheehan OC, Kyne L, Kelly A et al. Population—based study of ABCD2 score, carotid stenosis and atrial fibrillation for early stroke prediction after transient ischaemic attack. *Stroke* 2010;41:844-850.

45. Chandratheva A, Mehta Z, Geragthy OC et al Population-based study of risk and predictors of stroke in the first few hours after transient ischaemic attack. *Neurology* 2009;72:1941-1947.

46. Gommans J, Barker PA, Fink J. Preventing stroke: the assessment and management of people with transient ishaemic attack. *NZ Med J* 2009; 122(1293): 3856.

47. Rothwell PM, Giles MP, Chandratheva A et al. On behalf of the Early use of Existing Preventive Strategies for Stroke (EXPRESS) study. Effect of urgent

treatment of transient ischaemic attack and minor stroke on early recurrent stroke (EXPRESS) study: a prospective population based sequential comparison. *Lancet* 2007; 370: 1432-1442.

48. Lasserson DS. Initial management of suspected transient ischaemic attack and stroke in primary care: implications of recent research. *Postgrad Med J* 2009; 85(1003): 422-7.

49. Van de Griend JP, Saseen JJ. Combination of antiplatelet agents for the prevention of stroke. *Pharmacotherapy* 2008;28(0):1233-42.

50. Adams RJ, Albers G, Albert MJ et al. Update to the AHA/ASA Recommendations for the Prevention of Stroke in Patients With Stroke and Transient Ischaemic Attack. *Stroke* 2008;39:1647-1652

51. Diener HC, Cunha L, Forbes C. et al. European Stroke Prevention Study 2. dipyridamole and acetylsalicyclic acid in the secondary prevention of stroke (ESPS-2). *J Neuro Sci* 1993; 143 (1-2): 1-13.

52. Chaturvedi S. Acetylsalicyclic acid plus extended release combination therapy for secondary stroke prevention. *Clin Ther* 2008;30(7):1196-205 (abstract).

53. Kirshner HS. prevention of secondary stroke and TIA with antiplatelet therapy: the role of the primary care physician. *Int J Clin Pract* 2007;6 (10):1739-40 (abstract).

54. Cina C, Clase C, Haynes BR. Carotid endarterectomy for symptomatic carotid stenosis. In: *The Cochrane Library*, Issue 4. Oxford: Update Software; 2001.

11

CAROTID ARTERY DISEASE IN THE ELDERLY

Introduction

In the mid 1600s Johannes Jacob Wepfer a Swiss physician through autopsy studies traced the carotid and vertebral arteries from their origin in the aorta to the base of the brain. He recognized that stroke could result not only from bleeding in the brain but also from blockage of the vessels that supply the brain. Stroke is the most common neurological disorder and third leading cause of death in the adults[1]. Approximately 25% of the ischaemic strokes are due to embolism from the heart, 25% due to small vessel disease and the remainder to large vessel disease[2]. The incidence of symptomatic carotid stenosis increases with age. There is however a significant under investigation in routine clinical practice in patients aged more than 80 years with transient ischaemic attack or ischaemic stroke in spite of their willingness to have surgery[3]. The North American Carotid Endarterectomy Trial (NASCET)[4] and the European Carotid Surgery Trial (ECST)[5] have shown that screening for this disease in symptomatic patients has become singularly meaningful and evidence of considerable benefit from endarterectomy[5,6]. Imaging of the extracranial amd intracranial vasculature have become significant part of the evaluation of patients with stroke or TIA. The first carotid endarterectomy was performed in the 1950s.

Incidence prevalence epidemiology and risk factors

Extracranial carotid artery disease is the cause of stroke in 14-40% of patients and artery to artery embolism is the main mechanism of ischaemic stroke[7]. In a study of 307 patients over the age of 65 years referred to a vascular surgeon for reasons other than for cerebovascular disease revealed a prevalence of asymptomatic carotid artery stenosis of more than 70% in 27% of the patients [8]. Furthermore they were associated with male gender, diabetes mellitus, advanced age and had quitted smoking[8]. In order to assess prevalence a total of 6,727 persons aged 25-84 years were screened for extracranial

134

stenosis with Duplex ultrasound of the right carotid artery [9] and 225 persons were found to have carotid stenosis. The prevalence was higher in men (3.8%) compared to women (2.7%) and the carotid stenosis was significantly associated with coronary artery disease, peripheral artery disease and a history of cerebrovascular disease[9].

The association of carotid artery disease with coronary artery disease[10] peripheral vascular disease[11], atheromatous renal artery stenosis[12] aortic-iliac occlusive disease[13] and history of cerebrovascular disease is well documented. There is a high prevalence of significant internal carotid stenosis ranging from 1.3-8.5% in patients undergoing cardiac surgery[14,15]. However the yield of significant ICA stenosis (70% or more) which would benefit from carotid endarterectomy according to the Asymptomatic Carotid Surgery trial was found to be low in patients who had undergone previous coronary angioplasty[16]. The presence of carotid stenosis in the general population as measured by ultrasound was found to be low [9].

Patients undergoing aortic reconstruction are commonly found to have internal carotid artery (ICA) disease. ICA stenosis of more than 50% was found in 64 of 240 cases undergoing aortic reconstruction for aortic aneurysm and aortic-iliac occlusive disease and was much more common in the latter[13]. Four out of 10 patients with atheromatous renal artery stenosis severe enough to require angioplasty appeared to have moderate to severe carotid artery disease [12]. The prevalence of > or =50% carotid stenosis carotid territory events is lower than the prevalence of > or = 50% vertebral and basilar stenosis in posterior circulation TIA or minor stroke and is associated with multiple TIAs and a high risk of early recurrent stroke [17].

Age, male gender[3,8,9], total cholesterol[9,13], smoking[9] are all independent predictors of carotid artery disease. The Atheromatous Risk Community Study (The ARIC Study) (14,502 black and white middle-aged patients) demonstrated a prevalence of 30% with metabolic syndrome (MS)[18]. The study revealed subjects with MS are twice more likely to have prevalent coronary heart disease and greater carotid intimal-medial wall thickness after adjustment for age, gender and race[18]. The ARIC study found that Blacks have 6% thicker arterial walls at the level of the common carotid but no significant difference at the bifurcation or ICA[19,20]. The Insulin Resistance Atherosclerotic Study demonstrated similar results in Blacks and Whites and the Hispanics had 4-5% thinner arterial walls at the common carotid artery[21]. There are differences in the prevalence of symptomatic carotid stenosis between ethnicities. There are reports of higher prevalence of carotid stenosis in Blacks compared to White stroke patients[22]. Other investigators however have shown similar or slightly lower rates of stenosis between Blacks and Whites [21,23].

Pathophysiology

To appreciate what happens in stroke or TIA it is crucial to understand the mode of distribution of the blood vessels to the brain and the extracranial to-intracranial collateral pathways, the pial-to-pial collateral pathways and variabilities of the circle of Willis (Chapter 2). For instance, in ischaemic stroke leptomeningeal collaterals on CT angiography are reliable markers of good outcome[24]. The carotid artery can be involved by a number of different pathologies, atherosclerotic carotid artery disease, carotid artery stenosis, spontaneous carotid artery dissection, carotid artery tortuosity and kinking and atherosclerotic aortic arch disease, traumatic occlusion and inflammatory arteriopathies[25]. The ICA and ECA branches of the common carotid artery are the common sites for plaque formation in the cerebrovascular system. The carotid bifurcation and the proximal ICA are most frequently involved. The distal carotid artery and the origin of the middle cerebral artery and the carotid siphon may also be affected.

Atherosclerosis is one of the main risk factors for ischaemic stroke. Carotid artery disease results from atherosclerosis leading to plaque formation, plaque ulceration, narrowing of vessels in thromboembolism and carotid embolic disease. Shear stress and turbulent flow have been shown experimentally to increase endothelial permeability[26]. Insudation of lipoproteins mainly low density lipoproteins (LDL) into the intima results in fluid full foam cells, the hallmark of atherosclerosis. As the plaque evolves denudation of the endothelium occurs. As a result of endothelial injury a thrombogenic cascade is triggered. At the same time the coagulation cascade is initiated. Thrombi are formed over the plaque as a result of loss of endothelium where the thrombus forms on the surface and within the plaque as a result of plaque rupture. The plaques may undergo calcification, form fissured or ulcerated lesions and the ruptured plaque exposes highly thrombogenic substances which encourage thrombus formation or release of emboli into the blood stream[27] and obstruction to blood flow by increasing plaque burden (Chapter 4). Dense carotid calcification may be seen in the absence of high grade carotid stenosis and on the other hand high grade stenosis of the proximal carotid artery may occur in the absence of calcification. Fig.11.1 CT scan showing calcification in the ICA.

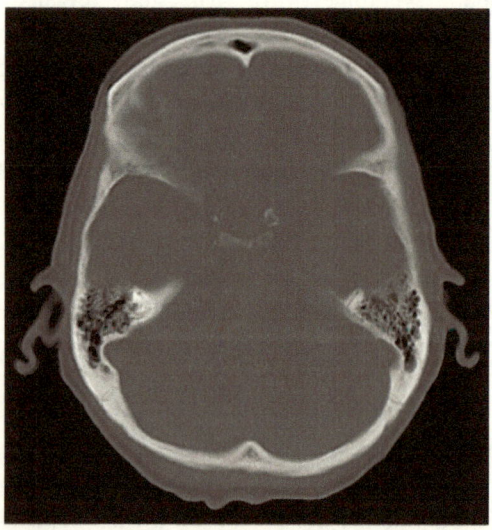

Fig 11.1 CT scan showing calcification in the ICA

White matter lesions are commonly seen on magnetic resonance images in the elderly and have been associated with motor, cognitive and psychiatric morbidity[28]. White matter lesions are divided into those in the periventricular and those in the subcortical region. It is well known that advanced age and hypertension are risk factors in the development white matter lesions. de Leeuw et al [29] in a population based study on the association of atherosclerosis in the carotid arteries and white matter lesions in subjects between 60-90 years found that greater the increase in the number of plaques in the carotid arteries the more severe were the periventricular white matter lesions but not in the case of subcortical white matter lesions.

Atherosclerotic disease of the aortic arch and stroke

Atherosclerotic disease of the aortic arch should be considered as a risk factor for ischaemic stroke and a possible source of cerebral emboli [30]. Aortic plaque is a manifestation of generalized atherosclerosis. Advancing age, hypertension, hypercholestraemia and smoking are the well known risk factors. Two studies found that the prevalence of severe aortic plaque in stroke patients were of the same significance as that of two other causes of embolic stroke namely, atrial fibrillation and carotid artery disease[30,31]. The risk of stroke in 1 year for patients with severe plaque in the aortic arch on TEE is between 10-12% [32]. Patients with protruding plaques or with notable complexity have a high risk of subsequent vascular events [33]. In recent years there is increasing evidence that besides embolism a compromised cerebral blood flow may contribute in causing TIA and stroke in patients with carotid artery occlusion. It can be surmised in this situation there could be failure of the collateral blood flow via the circle of Willis, the pial-pial-collaterals and the opthalamic artery.

Evaluation

The finding of an audible carotid bruit in an asymptomatic patient may be the first indication for further evaluation. Only about one-third of the patients with a carotid bruit have haemodynamically significant stenosis (70-90%). The determination of vessels which may be diseased is crucial for patient management especially if carotid endarterectomy is contemplated. A variety of imaging procedures are available relatively safe and reliable and each technique however has its usefulness and its shortcomings.

Carotid-Doppler Ultrasonography (C-DUS) is used to detect luminal narrowing based on the velocity of blood flow across a stenotic lesion and other structural details of the carotids[34]. Although it has high sensitivity and specificity for detecting significant stenosis of the internal carotid (ICA)[35] it is less so in determining stenosis less than 50%. Furthermore the intracranial part of the ICA cannot be evaluated. It is non-invasive and inexpensive but is operator dependent. When combined with MR angiography and transcranial doppler it may be an alternative to conventional angiography[35].

Transcranial Doppler (TCD) detects and quantifies intracranial vessel stenosis, occlusions, collateral flow, embolic events and cerebral vasospasm[36,37]. The cerebral vessels are insonated through several windows in the skull[38]. The transtemporal approach is used to insonate the major intracerebral vessels and the terminal internal carotid artery[39]. The transforaminal approach insonates the terminal vertebral arteries and the basilar artery. ICA siphon and ophthalmic artery are insonated via the transorbital approach[38,40]. TCD is capable of detecting microembolic signals originating from conditions which are associated with microemboli such as carotid stenosis, atrial fibrillation, patent foramen ovale, prosthetic heart valves and plaque in the aortic arch[34]. Together with C-DUS it provides information as to the collateral flow patterns in high grade carotid lesion [39]. It is painless, non-invasive, safe [34] and cheap and can be performed by portable machines.

Computed tomographic angiography (CTA) is found to have a high sensitivity and high negative predictive value for carotid disease. It appears to be an excellent screening test for ICA stenosis and was advocated to be included in the initial imaging of patients with acute ischaemic stroke[41]. Its accuracy for detecting intra-arterial thrombus is close to that of DSA[42] which remains the gold standard for detection of many types of cerebrovascular lesons and diseases[34]. Another study however found the tendency of CTA to over estimate the degree of stenosis[43].

Contrast material enhancer—*Magnetic Resonance Angiography (CE-MRA)* has good sensitivity for detecting high grade stenosis. It produces an image of the artery. It is expensive, time-consuming and not readily available.

Cerebral angiography, DSA is the gold standard for imaging the carotid arteries and it allows evaluation of the entire carotid artery system. It provides information about plaque morphology and collateral circulation. It is invasive, expensive and can cause serious complications such as stroke and death[34]. The degree of stenosis is determined with high degree of accuracy by CTA and DSA with the latter superior to CTA[34].

Carotid endarterectomy (CEA)

The optimal management of symptomatic and nonsymptomatic carotid disease remains debatable despite several trials and several years of research [44]. Based on studies the American Heart Association[45] recommends: A symptomatic ipsilateral carotid stenosis of 70-99% is a proven indication for carotid endarterectomy (CEA) provided the surgical risk does not exceed 6%. For symptomatic patients with 30-60% stenosis CEA is acceptable but has not been proven to be of benefit. For symptomatic patients with 0-29% stenosis CEA is not beneficial.

Asymptomatic patients with stenosis 60-99% are considered to have a proven indication for CEA provided the surgical risk is less than 3% and life expectancy is not less than 5 years[45]. The benefit/risk ratio is smaller in this group compared to symptomatic patients and decisions must be individualized[46]. Data from a 10-year follow up the Asymptomatic Carotid Surgery Trail did not show any significant change in the absolute risk reduction from stroke or operative death compared to best medical treatment[47].

Best medical treatment includes statins, antiplatelet therapy and treatment of blood pressure in symptomatic patients[48,49]. In the NASCET elderly patients over 75 years of age with symptomatic carotid stenosis gained the most relative stroke reduction from CEA versus medical therapy[50]. There is now increasing evidence that the risk of stroke in patients with asymptomatic carotid artery stenosis on medical treatment alone has fallen[51] to about 2% per annum[47]. Medical treatment alone is now considered the best treatment for asymptomatic carotid artery stenosis[52] except in those patients who are at risk of stroke. According to Cardona et al [53] CEA with best medical treatment might be better than medical management alone or surgery in preventing stroke.

Reports on peri-procedural outcome in patients over the age of 80 years following carotid vascularization are conflicting[54]. According to Reichmann et al [54] the major adverse event rates after CEA in octogenarians were comparable to results of large randomized trials in younger patients. In another study in patients aged 80 or more the combined stroke and death rate fell within acceptable levels and compared favourably with best medical care[55]. There are other reports of greater rates of perioperative mortality and morbidity with CEA in nonagenarians compared to younger patients including octagenarians[56]. Hingorani et al [57] compared three groups, 53-79 year old, 80-89 year old and 90-98 year old patients who had had CEA. They found the perioperative death and stroke rate were 1.8% vs 2.1% vs 10% respectively. In general, patients over 80 years old should not be arbitrarily considered as 'high risk for CEA[54,55].

Percutaneous transluminal carotid angioplasty and carotid stents

Age is a risk factor for CEA especially in those 80 years and over. Carotid artery stenting (CAS) frequently with filter devices has emerged as an alternative to carotid endarterectomy (CEA) for treating carotid stenosis. However, there is an increasing risk of perioperative stroke and death with CAS with increasing age and treatment within two weeks of neurological symptoms in symptomatic patients[58]. Severity of the lesion, calcification, aortic arch elongation, tortuosity, and great vessel origin stenosis together with the combined perioperative stroke/myocardial infarction/ death rate was 10.8% in the subgroup of patients for CAS in their 80s[59]. CAS is also associated with increased peri-procedural complications[60]. Despite the use of distal protection devices CAS is associated with a higher burden of microemboli compared to CEA[61]. In a single center review of CAS performed on 24 patients over the age of 80 years (range 80-91) and 16 men (70.8%) were symptomatic the success rate was 100% with residual stenosis of <20%. At one follow up there were no deaths as well as no re-stenosis[60]. The International Carotid Stenting Study reported a 2-fold higher procedural risk of stroke in the endovascular group and a five-fold increase in new infarcts on DWMR imaging[62]. The North American Carotid Revascularisation Endarterectomy vs Stenting Trial (CREST) showed similar rates though non significant, of stroke, myocardial infarction and death in its endarterectomy and stenting groups in the periprocedural period and at 4 years[63]. The SPACE Trail reported higher re-stenosis following stenting [64]. Of the 142 consecutive patients aged 80 years and over who underwent stenting 72% were asymptomatic a 30-day rate of stroke and death was 3.3%, 2.6% in the asymptomatic patients and 5.1% in the symptomatic[65]. Recent data suggest that cognitive function may decline after CEA and the two mechanisms for cognitive decline are emboli and hypoperfusion [61]. Embolic events during CAS might be greater than observed during CEA [66,67].

Patients with complete occlusion of the carotid artery, previous stroke with dense neurological deficit, severe comorbidity and those with a haemorrhagic component to their stroke are excluded from CEA. There is a variable risk of stroke or death in the perioperative period. Cardiac events are the most common cause of mortality and hence pertinent preoperative workup is crucial. In a trial in which surgeons were carefully selected the permanent disabling stroke and death rate was 2.3% and the rate of peri-operative stroke and death wa 5.3%[68]. In patients undergoing CEA the following are recognized as predictors of adverse events: age above 75 years, symptoms status, severe hypertension, angina, evidence of ICA thrombus or stenosis near the carotid siphon and endarterectomy performed in preparation for coronary bypass surgery[69]. Perioperative stroke was clearly technically related in 65% of the cases and unrelated to patient's age, sex or associated problems[70]. Technical failure would be enhanced by the presence of hypertension, preoperative neurological deficits and contralateral carotid occlusion resulting in perioperative stroke[71].

Two types of periendartectomy strokes have been described. One with water shed patterns with varied symptomatology and the other with territorial infarction with a hemispheric syndrome[72]. Haemodynamic insufficiency during clamping of the carotid artery or thromboembolism could be the mechanisms of functional damage during CEA. There may be others that could contribute to the topographical localization and symptomatology, namely cerebral dysautoregulation, transhemispheric diachiasis, variations in the arterial tree, collateral flow and deep perforators from the carotid system. TCD has demonstrated embolic signals during the dissection phase of carotid endarterectomy[73]. Jansen et al[73] emphasized that microemboli into haemodynamically compromised area will contribute to the ischaemia in the territory with the lowest perfusion that is, the watershed areas.

Thrombolysis or mechanical recanalisation has been used to restore blood flow following acute ischaemic stroke. In some patients reperfusion gives rise to cerebral reperfusion injury resulting in oedema and haemorrhage and this can occur as a complication of carotid endarterectomy or intracranial stenting. Several mechanisms have been proposed in the pathogenesis of reperfusion injury such as dysautoregulation.

CLINICAL RELEVANCE-Carotid artery disease

* Approximately 50% of the ischaemic strokes are due to large vessel disease.
* The incidence of symptomatic carotid stenosis increases with age.
* Carotid artery disease results from atherosclerosis leading to plaque formation, plaque ulceration, narrowing of vessels in thromboembolism and carotid embolic disease.
* The association of carotid artery disease with coronary artery disease, peripheral vascular disease, atheromatous renal artery stenosis, aorto-iliac occlusive disease and a history of cerebrovascular disease is well documented.
* There is however a significant under investigation in routine clinical practice in patients aged more than 80 years with transient ischaemic attack or ischaemic stroke in spite of their willingness to have surgery.
* Imaging of the extra and intracranial vasculature have become significant part of the evaluation of patients with stroke or TIA.
* The degree of stenosis can be determined with high degree of accuracy by CTA or DSA with the latter superior to CTA.
* A symptomatic ipsilateral carotid stenosis of 70-99% is a proven indication for carotid endarterectomy (CEA) provided the surgical risk does not exceed 6%. For symptomatic patients with 30-60% stenosis CEA is acceptable but has not been proven to be of benefit[45]. Plaque morphology may be a factor. For symptomatic patients with 0-29% stenosis CEA is not beneficial[45].
* Asymptomatic patients with stenosis 60-99% are considered to have a proven indication for CEA provided the surgical risk is less than 3% and life expectancy is not less than 5 years[45].
* Atherosclerotic disease of the aortic arch should be considered as a risk factor for ischaemic stroke and possible source of emboli[30].
* Patients over 80 years old should not be arbitrarily considered as 'high risk for CEA[54,55].
* Medical treatment alone is now considered the best treatment for asymptomatic carotid artery stenosis except in those patients who are at risk of stroke[52].
* Best medical treatment includes statins, antiplatelet therapy and treatment of blood pressure.
* Cognitive function may decline after CEA and the two mechanisms for cognitive decline are emboli and hypoperfusion[61].
* Embolic events during CAS might be greater than observed during CEA[66,67].
* Several mechanisms such as dysautoregulation has been proposed in the pathogenesis of reperfusion injury which can occur after CEA and CAS.

REFERENCES

1. WHO-Stroke 1989. Recommendations on prevalence, diagnosis and therapy: report of the WHO task force in stroke and other cerebrovascular disorders. *Stroke* 1989; 20: 1407-1431.
2. van Gijn J. Main groups of cerebral and spinal vascular diseases: overview. In Ginsberg MD, Bogousslasky J eds. Cerebrovascular disease, pathophysiology, diagnosis and management Malden. Mass. Blackwell, Science, 1998; 1369-1372.
3. Fairhead JF, Rothwell PM. Underinvestigation and undertreatment of carotid disease in elderly patients with transient ischaemic attack and stoke: a comparative population-based study. *Brit Med J* 2006; 333(7567): S25-7.
4. North American Carotid Endarterectomy Trial (NASCET) Collaborators. Beneficial effect of carotid endarterectomy in symptomatic patients with high grade stenosis. *N Engl J Med* 1998; 339: 1415-1425.
5. European Carotid Surgery Trial (ECST) collaborators group. Randomized trial of endarterectomy for recently symptomatic carotid stenosis: final results of the MRC European Carotid Surgery trial. *Lancet* 2004; 363: 1491-1502.
6. Barnett HJ, Taylor DW, Eliasz WM et al. Benefits of carotid endarterectomy in patients with symptomatic moderate to severe stenosis. North American Symptomatic Carotid Endarterectomy Trial Collaborators. *New Engl J Med* 1998; 339: 1415-1425 [abstract].
7. Niesen WD, Sliwka U, Lingnan A, Noth J. Cerebral emboli in cryptogenic ischaemia: a reason to enforce diagnostic testing. *J Stroke Cerebrovasc* 2001; 10: 44-48.
8. Ascher E, DePippo P, Salles-Cunha S et al. Carotid screening with duplex ultrasound in elderly asymptomatic patients referred to vascular surgery. *Ann Vasc Surg* 2009; 13: 164-168 [abstract].
9. Mathiesen EB, Joakinsen O, Benoa KH. Prevalence of and risk factors associated with carotid artery stenosis: The Tromse Study. *Cerebrovasc Dis* 2001; 12: 44-51.
10. Touboul PJ, Elbaz A, Koller C et al. On behalf of the GENIC investigators. Common carotid artery intima-media thickness and ischemic stroke: the GENIC case-control study. *Circulation* 2000; 02: 313-318.
11. Ahmed B, Al-Karaffof H. Prevalence of significant asymptomatic carotid artery disease in patients with peripheral vascular disease: a meta—analysis. *Eur J Vasc endovasc Surg* 2009; 37: 261-271.
12. Missouris C, Papavassiliou M, Khaw K et al. High prevalence of carotid artery stenosis. *Nephrology Dialysis Transplant* 1998; 13: 945-948.
13. Cahan A, Killewich LA, Kolodner L. The prevalence of carotid artery stenosis inpatients undergoing aortic reconstruction. *Am J Surg* 1999; 178: 182-231.

14. Solasides GC, Latter D, Steinmetz OK et al. Carotid endartectomy duplex scanning in pre-operatiive assessment for coronary artery vasculaization. *J Vasc Surg* 1995; 21: 359-364.

15. Meharwal ZS, Mishra A, Trehan N. Safety and efficiency of one stage off-pump coronary artery operation and carotid endarterectomy. *Ann Thoracic Surg* 2002; 73: 793-97.

16. Fassiadis N, Adams K, Zayed H et al. Occult carotids artery disease in patients who have undergone coronary angioplasty. *Interact Cardiovasc Thorac Surg* 2000; 7: 855-857.

17. Marquardt L, Kuer W, Chandratheva A et al. Incidence and prognosis of > or 50% symptomatic vertebral or basilar artery stenosis: prospective population—based study. *Brain* 2009; 132: 982-8.

18. McNeill AM, Rosamund WD, Girmen CJ et l. Prevalence of coronary heart disease—carotid artery thickening in patients with metabolic syndrome (the ARIC study). *Am J Cardiol* 2004; 15: 1249-54.

19. Folon AC, Eckfeldt JH, Weitznan S et l. Relation of carotid artery wall thickness in diabetics mellitus, fasting glucose insulin body size and physical activity. *Stroke* 1991; 75: 66-73.

20. Burke GI, Evans GW, Hutchinson R et al. Racial differences on carotid artery wall thickness in middle-aged adults. *Circulation* 1990; 89: 939.(abstract).

21. Howard G, O'Leary DH, Zaccard D et al. Insulin sensitivity and atherosclerosis. *Circulation* 1996; 93: 1808-1817.

22. McGarry P, Serberg LA, Guzonan M. Cerebral atherosclerosis in New Orleans. *Lab Invest* 1985; 52: 533-539.

23. Ryu JE, Murros K, Espeland MA et al. Extracranial carotid atherosclerosis on black and white patients with transient ischaemic attacks. *Stroke* 1989; 20: 1133-1137.

24. Lima FO, Furie KL, Silva GS et al. The pattern of leptomeningeal collaterals on CT angiography is a strong predictor of long term functional outcome in stroke patients with large vessel intracranial occlusion. *Stroke* 2010; 41: 2316-2322.

25. Graham AM, Moore WS, Baker W. Carotid artery disease. website: *http:// updvs.vascular* webng/APDVS_contribution_Pages Curriculum/clinical/os-carotid accessed 20/03/2010.

26. Kumar V, Contran RS, Robbins SL. Basic Pathology. Fifth Ed. WR Saunders Co, Philadelphia 1992.

27. Hogan N, Boenau I. Transient ishaemic attack. *Emerg Med* 2006; 38: 41-46.

28. TaylorWD, MacFall JR, Provenzak, JM et al. Serial MR imaging volumes of hyperintense white matter lesions in elderly patients:Correlation with vascular risk factors. *AJR* 2003;180:571-576.

29. de Leeuw FE, de Groot JC, Bots ML et al. Carotid atherosclerosis and cerebral white matter lesions in a population based magnetic resonance imaging study. *J Neurol* 2000;247:291-296.

30. Amarenco P, Cohen A, Tzourio C et al. Atherosclerotic disease of the aortic arch and the risk of ischaemic stroke. *N Engl J Med* 1994; 331: 1474-1479.

31. Jones EF, Kalnran JM, Calafiore D. Proximal aortic atheroma: an independent risk factor for cerebral ischaemic attacks. *Stroke* 1995; 26: 218-224.

32. Kronzon T, Tunich PA. Aortic atherosclerotic disease in stroke. *Circulation* 2006; 114: 63-75.

33. Mitsch R, Doherty C, Wircherfening H et al. Vascular events during follow up in patients with aortic arch atherosclerosis. *Stroke* 1997; 28: 36-39.

34. Latchaw RE, Alberts MJ, Lev MH et al. Recommendations for imaging of acute ischaemic stroke. A scientific statement from the American Heart Association. *Stroke* 2009; 40: 3646-3678.

35. Suwanwela N, Can U, Furrie KL. Et al. Carotid Doppler ultrasound criteria for internal carotid artery stenosis based on residual lumen diameter calculated from en block carotid endarterecromy specimens. *Stroke* 1996;27: 1965-1969.

36. Newill DW, Aaslid R. Transcranial Doppler—clinical and exprerimental uses. *Cerebrovasc Brain Metab Rev* 1992; 4: 1222-143.

37. Babikian VL, Pocjhav V, Burdette DE., Brass ML. Transcranial Doppler sonographic monitoring in the intensive care unit. *J Intensive care Med* 1991;6:

38. Fujoka KA, Donville CM. Anatomy free hand examination technique. In Newill DW, Aaslid R.eds *Transcranial Doppler*. New York Raven.1992

39. Markus HS. Transcranial Doppler ultrasound. Brit Med Bull 2000;56(2): 378-388.

40. Alexandrov AV, Sloan MA, Wong LK et al. Practical standards for transcranial Doppler, ultrasound. Part 1-Test performance. *J Neurosurgery* 2007; 117: 11-18.

41. Josephson SA, Bryant S O, Johnston SC et al. Evaluation of carotid stenosis using CT angiography in initial evaluation of stroke and transientischaemic attack. *Neurology* 2004; 63: 457-460.

42. Lev MH, Farkas J, Rodriguez VR. et al CT angiography in the rapid triage of patients with hyperacute stroke to intraarterial thrombolysis: accuracy in the detection of large vessel thrombus. *J Comput Assist Tomogr* 2001; 25: 520-528.

43. Feasby TE, Findlay JM. CT angiography for the assessment of carotid stenosis. *Neurology* 2004; 63: 412-43.

44. Lovrencic-Huzjan A, Rundek T, Katsnelson M. Recommendations for management of patients with carotid stenosis. *Stroke Res Treat* 2012;2012: 175869: doi 10:1155/2012/175869. Epub 2012 May 7 (abstract)

45. Americam Heart Association. Guidelines for carotid endarterectomy. A statement for health care professionals for a special working group of stroke Council. *Circulation* 1998: 97: 501.

46. Chatuvedi S, Bruno A, Feasby T et al. Carotid endarterectomy-an evidence—based review: report of Therapeutics and Technology Assessment Subcommittee of the American Academy of Neurology. *Neurology* 2005;65(6):794-801 (abstract).

47. Halliday A, Mandfield A, Marro J et al. Prevention of disabling and fatal strokes by successful carotid endarterectomy in patients with recent neurological symptoms: randomized controlled trial. *Lancet* 2004; 363: 1491-1502.

48. Ederie J, Brown MM. The evidence for medicine versus surgery for carotid stenosis. *Eur J Radiol* 2006;60(1):3-7 (abstract)

49. Kassaian SE, Goodarzynejad H. Carotid artery stenting, enarterectomy or medical treatment: the debate is not over. *J Tehran Heart Cent* 2011; 6(1):1-13 (abstract)

50. Alamnowitch S, Eliasziw M, Meldrum H, Barnett HIM. Risk causes and prevention of ischaemic stroke in elfderly patients with symptomatic carotid-artery stenosis. *Lancet* 2001;357: 1154-1160 (abstract).

51. Marquardt L, Geraghty OC, Mehta Z et al. Low risk of ipsilateral stroke inpatients with asymptomatic carotid stenosis on best medical treatment: prospective population based strudy. *Stroke* 2009; 2010; 41.

52. Abbott A. Medical (nonsurgical) intervention alone is now best for prevention of stroke associated with asymptomatc severe carotid stenosis: results of a systemic review and analysis. *Stroke* 2009;40:e573-e583.

53. Cardona P, Rubio F, Martinez-Yelamos S, Krupinski J. Endarterectomy, best medical treatment or both for stroke prevention in patients with asymptomatic carotid artery stenosis. Cerebrovasc Dis 2007;24(Suppl 1):126-33 (abstract).

54. Reichmann BL, van Lammeren GW, Moll FL, de Borst GJ. Is age of 80 years a threshold for carotid vascularization? *Curr Cardiol Res* 2011;7(1):15-21 (abstract).

55. Miller MT, Comerata AJ, Tzilinis A. et al. Carotid endarterectomy in octogenarians: does increased age indicate 'high risk?'. *J Vasc Surg* 2005;41(2):231-7 (abstract).

56. Teso D, Edwards RE, Frattini JC et al. Safety of carotid enartectomy in 2,443 elderly patients: lessons from nonagenarians—are we pushing the limit? *J Am Coll Surg* 2005;200(5):734-741.

57. Hingorani A, Ascher E, Schutzer R et al. Carotid endarterectomy in octagenarians and nonagenarians: is it worth the effort. Acta Chir Belg 2004;104(4):384-7.

58. Topakian R, Strasak AM, Sonnberger M et al. Timing of stenting of symptomatic carotid stenosis is predictive of 30-day outcome. *Eur J Neurol* 2007; 14: 672-678.

59. Lam RC, Lin SC, DeRoberts B. et al. The impact of increasing age on anatomic fasctors affecting carotid angioplasty and stenting. *J Vasc Surg* 2007; 45: 875-880.

60. Linfante I, Andreone V, Akkawi N, Wakhloo AK. Internal carotid artery stenting in patients over the age of 80 years: single center experience and review of the literature. *J Neuroimaging* 2009; 19(2): 158-63 (abstract).

61. Ghogawala Z, Westerveld M, Amin-Hanjani S. Cognitive outcomes after revascularisation: the role of cerebral emboli and hypoperfusion. *Neurosurgery* 2008;62: 385-395(abstract).

62. Brown MM, Ederle J, Bonati LH. Safety results of the International Carotid Stenting Study: Early outcome of patients randomized between carotid stenting and endarterectomy for symptomatic carotid stenosis. European Stroke Conference. 2009. Stockholm, Sweden. May 26-29,2009.

63. Brott TG, Hobson RW 2nd, Howard G et al. Stenting versus endarterectomy for treatment of carotid-artery stenosis. *N Engl J Med* 2010; 363: 11-23.

64. Eckstein HH, Ringleb P, Allenberg JR. et al. Results of the Stent-Protected Angioplasty versus Carotid Endarterectomy (SPACE) study to treat symptomatic stenoses at 2 years: a multinational, prospective, randomized trial. *Lancet Neurol* 2008; 7: 893-902.

65. Chiam PT, Roubin GS, Panagoppulos G et al. One-year clinical outcomes mid-term survival and predictors of mortality after carotid stenting in elderly patiernts. *Circulation* 2009;119:2343-2348.

66. Crawley F, Stygall J, Lunn S et al. Comparison of microembolism detetected by transcranial Doppler and neuropsychological sequelae of carotid surgery asnd percutaneous transluminal angioplasty. *Stroke* 200;31:1329-1334.

67. Ilhara K, Murao K, Sakai N. et al. Outcome of carotid endarterectomy and stent insertion based on grading of carotid enarterectomy risk: A 7-year prospective study. *J Neurosurg* 2006;105:546-554.

68. Reinmulh UM, Dyken ML. Carotid endarterectomy, bright light at the end of the tunnel. *Stroke* 1991; 2: 200-15.

69. McCroy DC, Goldstein LB, Samsa GP et al. Predicting complications of carotid endarterectomy. *Stroke* 1993;24:1285-91.

70. Riles TS, Imparato AM, Jacobowitz GR et al. The cause of perioperative stroke after carotid endarterectomy. *J Vasc Surg* 1994;19:206-16.

71. Nagaratnam N, Kalouche H, Chen E, Grice D. Clinical-CT correlations following periendareretomy stroke. *Eur J Int Med* 1997; 8: 201-204.

72. Jansen C, Ramos LMP, Van Heeswijk et al. Impact of microembolism and haemodynamic changes in the brain during carotid endarterectomy. *Stroke* 1994; 25: 992-97.

12

CLINICAL SYNDROMES RELATED

TO CAROTID ARTERY DISEASE

1. Transient ischaemic attack/Transient monocular blindness
2. Dissection of the carotid artery
3. Vertebro-basilar steal and carotid artery stenosis
4. Ocular ischaemic syndrome
5. Shaking limb syndrome
6. Carotid stenosis in vascular cognitive impairment
7. Kinks coils and tortuosity of the carotid artery
8. Traumatic occlusion of the carotid artery

1. Transient ischaemic attack (TIA)/transient monocular blindness (TMB) have been described in Chapter 8.

2. Internal carotid artery dissection (ICAD)

Although a more common cause of stroke in the young and middle aged adult it can occur in older adults. The tear can either begin in the intima of the carotid artery or directly within the media, the blood dissecting along the artery to form an intramural haematoma. This may cause narrowing of the artery and a higher risk for thrombosis and embolization. The dissecting plane at times can be between the media and the adventitia causing an aneurymal dilatation which can cause mass effect and also be a site for emboli formation[1]. The cause for the dissection is unclear and it is generally accepted that dissection of the carotid artery is a multifactorial disease[1].

3. Vertebro-basilar steal and carotid artery stenosis

Internal carotid artery occlusion or high stenosis without vertebral and subclavian atherosclerosis can present with vertebro-basilar insufficiency (VBI)[2]. Bougousslavasky and Regli[2] found that greater size of visible infarct combined with weak collateral circulation and bilateral atherosclerosis of the ICA were associated with the occurrence of VBI. In another study the two patients described had severe carotid artery stenosis with 'steal VBI' and well developed collaterals through the ipsilateral posterior communicating artery and no occlusive disease of the vertebro-basilar system[3]. Blood flow studies revealed impaired haemodynamics in the contralateral occipital lobe which correlated with their neurological deficit. In both reports the symptoms improved with carotid endarterectomy and carotid stenting respectively and in the second report neurological improvement. The vertebrobasilar insufficiency in all probability is due to an intracranial steal from the vertebrobasilar system towards the carotid system.

4. Ocular ischaemic syndrome

Transient monocular blindness (TMB) or amaurosis fugax is a form of acute visual loss due to embolic material in the retinal arterioles. It lasts only for a few seconds or minutes with complete restoration of blood flow and retinal function. Severe chronic arterial hypotension to the eye gives rise to a spectrum of findings with progressive pathological changes. Severe unilateral or bilateral carotid artery stenosis or occlusion is the most common cause of the ocular ischaemic syndrome (OIS). Other causes are giant cell arteritis (GCA) and aortic arch syndrome. OIS occurs only when the carotid artery stenosis is severe, more than 90% [4]. Ischaemic changes consist of microaneurysms, mid—peripheral dot and blot haemorrhages and an occasional splinter haemorrhage[5]. As the disease progresses the anterior segment is involved and is then referred to as 'ischaemic oculopathy'[5]. At this stage visual function is normal. As the disease progresses vision becomes impaired.

In ischaemic retinopathy the most important finding is the neovascularization of the iris and angle with neovascular glaucoma (NVG)[5]. Intraocular pressure may rise and optic atrophy may develop and an incidental finding of cholesterol emboli (Hollenhorst plaques). Iris neovacularization has been found in up to 90% of patients and dilated episcleral vessels in 20%[6,7]. Spontaneous or easily inducible retinal artery pulsation is present in most cases and seen close to the disc[7].

OIS usually occurs between ages 50 and 80 years and men are afflicted twice as commonly as women. Most of the patients present with decreased vision and about half with eye pain. Ocular pain or discomfort around the orbit in the absence of glaucoma is seen in 5-10% of patients with OIS [7]. Occasionally bright light may precipitate vision loss ('bright light amaurosis') with subjective after-images of visual fragmentation, distortion or blurring [4]. Vision loss may also occur with change of posture or exertion [8,9]. There may be prior history of a TIA or TMB or often an association with system morbidity such as hypertension (50-73%), diabetes (56%), ischaemic heart disease (38-48%), stroke (27-31%) or peripheral vascular disease [6,10]. OIS can cause severe blindness and is due to occlusion of the internal carotid or common carotid arteries. Early diagnosis is crucial reducing the risk of ocular complications and future ischaemic heart disease and cerebrovascular disease.

Hypotensive retinopathy can mimick diabetic retinopathy but the latter is seldom unilateral (80%). In giant cell arteritis (GCA) the erythrocyte sedimentation rate may be elevated and the patient must be referred to the neurologist for management. Neovascularisation of the iris, retina or optic nerve is treated with panretinal photocoagulation[4]. The intraocular pressure reduced by topical medications—topical beta adrenergic antagonists, topical steroids and cylcoplegics along with carbonic anhydrase inhibitors.

Carotid endarterectomy is effective in improving or preventing the progress of OIS caused by ICA stenosis[11]. Carotid artery stenting was effective in improving ocular circulation and also improved chronic OIS caused by severe carotid artery stenosis [12]. If there is carotid stenosis 70-99% carotid endarterectomy has shown benefit in patients with an disabling stroke, TMB or TIA. By pass surgery (superficial temporal artery-middle cerebral artery) has been advocated if lesions are unresectable by carotid endarterectomy [4].

5. The shaking limb

Unilateral involuntary movements or shaking limb are known to occur with transient cerebral ischaemia as a manifestation of of severe stenosis or occlusion of the internal carotid artery. The movements usually last for a few minutes and is accompanied by weakness of the affected limb. Nagaratnam et al[14] described a patient with limb movements lasting for three days. It is frequently precipitated by rising from a chair or bed or hyperextending the neck, exercise or exertion[13;14]. This has been attributed to haemodynamic compromise. Furthermore diminished cerebral blood flow has been documented [15] and symptoms may cease following endarterectomy[16,17,18].

Many such patients have small infarcts on computed tomography (CT) in the appropriate hemisphere[13,17,19]. The accepted concept is that in TIA focal ischaemia is not accompanied by infarction although there is evidence to the contrary[20]. Magnetic resonance imaging (MRI) especially diffusion-weighted magnetic resonance has demonstrated that in one third of the patients with proven TIA have ischaemic changes. Electroencephalogram (EEG) usually shows slowed activity but no epiletiform patterns[13,17]. Lacunar infarctions have been known to occur with TIA or RIND and limb shaking should be included in the group of lacunar syndromes. Hemiballism has been included in the group of lacunar syndromes[16] and has been related to lacunar infarcts in the subthalmic nucleus[21]. A reversible hemiballism has been described with a lacunar infarct in the contralateral lenticular nucleus and documented on the CT scan[22].

6. Carotid artery stenosis and vascular cognitive impairment

There had been two longitudinal studies that suggested that atherosclerotic diseases are a risk factor for cognitive decline[23,24]. Whether cognitive function can be altered by chronic cerebral ischaemia associated with carotid artery stenosis remains unclear[25,26]. Rao[26] studied four groups of patients with age of 65 years and over with symptomatic carotid stenosis of >75%, first anterior circulation stroke, with peripheral vascular disease and healthy controls. The study revealed that patients with symptomatic carotid stenosis had a greater global impairment on CAMCOG and more severe impairtment in frontal lobe function than controls. In the Rotterdam study individuals aged 74 to 94 years with plaques in the carotid bifurcation were significantly associated with low MMSE scores and when compared this was not significant in individuals aged 50-64 years[27;28].

It is well documented that occlusion of the ICAs can cause dementia either by multifocal infarction or less commonly by haemodynamic mechanisms [29]. Tatemichi et al [29] described a patient with bilateral ICA and unilateral vertebral artery occlusions who presented with profound behavioural and cognitive change and the neuropsychological finding was consistent with dementia. After extracranial and intracranial cerebral bypass surgery his neuropsychological and behavioural impairment had improved. There are several studies that suggest the cognitive function improves in some patients after endarterectomy [30] and recently after stenting[31] but there are also reports to the contrary [32].

Johnston et al[33] documented that asymptomatic high grade stenosis of the left internal carotid artery was associated with cognitive impairment and decline and this effect did persist after adjustment for right—sided stenosis indicating the association is not due to underlying vascular risk factors or atherosclerosis in general.

Bakker et al[34] in their study of patients with carotid artery occlusion and ipsilateral transient ischaemic attacks found neither the presence of any vascular factor, the side of the symptomatic carotid occlusion, the uni-or bilaterality of the carotid occlusion nor the number of cerebral ischaemic lesions were predictors of cognitive impairment.

There is now considerable evidence to suggest that cognitive function may decline after carotid endarterectomy (CEA). Microemboli are often found in patients with atherosclerosis especially of the carotid arteries, aortic arch and with heart disease. Microemboli may be the cause of cognitive impairment. The mechanisms of functional damage during carotid endarerectomy include the detrimental effect of procedural emboli. Carotid artery stenting as an alternative to carotid endarterectomy is also associated with higher burden of microemboli despite the use of distal protection devices [35].

7. Coils, kinks and tortuosity of the carotid artery

Elongation of the carotid can manifest as coil, loop, kink or increased tortuosity. There has been several reports following the first report of kinking by Riser et al in 1951 [36]. Despite this the clinical relationship between these carotid abnormalities and cerebrovascular disease remains unclear.

It is not known what the incidence of coiling and kinking of the carotid artery is in the general population[37]. In the literature however the incidence varied between 10-58%[37,38]. In a study of 2453 angiogram in 1438 patients colinig of the ICA was observed in 88 (6%) and kinking in 65 (5%)[39]. Carotid tortuosity has been reported to be more common in the elderly (>60 years) and more in women than in men [40]. Other investigators however has found no significant gender differences, was equal or slightly greater in men [37,41].

Loops and coils have a developmental basis and by themselves do not cause cerebrovascular ischaemic arttacks[42]. Atherosclerosis, hypertension and ageing may play a part in the development of the carotid abnormalities but it appears ageing is more important risk than atherosclerosis[43]. Coiling is rare and is largely asymptomatic. Narrowing of the lumen due to coiling of the carotid artery can lead to turbulent blood flow, subintimal ulceration and embolization and manifest as a stroke or transient ischemic attack[44]. However the prevalence and location of haemodynamically significant lesions in patients with carotid tortuosity is relatively unknown[40]. All tortuous vessels with haemodynamically significant internal carotid artery disease the location of maximum stenosis was in the region before the angulation[40].

Coiling or to a lesser extent kinking can present as a pulsatile mass at the bifurcation or at the base of the neck. Angioplasty of the carotid bifurcation, endarterectomy, bypass graft and resection and anastomosis of the carotid artery, and dilatation of the dysplastic lesions were performed in 166 patients with stenotic coiling and kinking of the ICA[45]. The stenotic coiling or kinking was isolated in 20.1% of the patients and in 79.9% it was associated with other lesions of the ICA[45]. At a 5-year follow-up the actual survival was 80.97%, patency 96.12% and ipsilateral stroke-free rate was 93.12%[45].

8. Traumatic injury to neck and carotid occlusion

Internal carotid artery thrombosis can follow head and neck trauma. Despite the numerous reports the diagnosis is often delayed. This largely due to lack of awareness and to the delay in the development of signs and symptoms.

The incidence of carotid artery stenosis reported after blunt injury is 0.25% among 5825 persons[46]. Several types of injury causing carotid artery thrombosis such as injury to face and neck as a result of a fall[47,48], struck by a volley ball[47] sports diving [49], karate punch[50] and roller coaster ride[51] have been reported. Traumatic occlusion of the common carotid artery are not that common as ICA[52]. It is associated with a high mortality and morbidity[46,52].

Different syndromes have been recognized. i. There may be almost complete absence of neurological symptoms. ii. At the other extreme there is a rapid onset following the injury with symptoms of a massive contralateral hemiplegia and may be accompanied by sensory deficits of the cortical type and aphasia of the dominant hemisphere. Stroke in these patients is believed to be due to occlusive thromboembolism. One of the cases described by Yamaura et al[48] the patient following blows to the face came in 3 hours later with left hemiparesis. The carotid angiogram showed a tapered occlusion in the right cervical ICA. and the CT scan demonstrated a large cerebral infarction in the right cerebral hemisphere. The patient died 10 days later. iii. An important mode of presentation is a gradual developing contralateral hemiplegia[47].

CLINICAL RELEVANCE—
CAROTID ARTERY RELATED CLINICAL SYNDROMES

* ICA occlusion or high stenosis wthout vertebral or subclavian atherosclerosis can present with a vertebro-basilar insufficieny- 'steal VBI' and improves with carotid endarterectomy or stenting.

* Severe chronic hypotension from unilateral or bilateral carotid artery stenosis or occlusion is the commonest cause of ocular ischaemic syndrome.

* Shaking limb is known to occur with transient cerebral ischaemia and a manifestation of severe stenosis of the ICA.

* Cognitive impairment can be associated with carotid artery stenosis.

* Elongation of the carotid artery can manifest as coil, loop, kink or increased tortuosity.

* Carotid artery thrombosis can occur after injury to the face or neck.

REFERENCES

1. Zohrabian AD. Dissection, carotid artery *http://emedicine.mediscape.com/article/75* 906-overview.
2. Bogousslavsky J, Regli F. Vertebrobasilar transient ischaemic attacks in internal carotid artery occlusion or tight stenosis. *Arch Neurol* 1985; 42(1): 64-68 (abstract).
3. Schichinohe H, Kuroda S, Honkin K et al. Two cases of 'steal VBI' with stenosis of the internal carotid artery. *No Shinhei Gaka* 2001; 29(9): 811-6 (abstract).
4. Malhotra R, Gregory-Evans K. Management of ocular ischaemic syndrome. *Br J Opthalmol* 2000; 84: 1428-1431.
5. Carter JE. Chronic ocular ischamia and carotid vascular disease *Stroke* 1985; 16: 721-728.
6. Mizener JB, Podhajsky P, Hayreh SC. Ocular Ischaemic Syndrome *Opthalmology* 1997; 104: 859-64.
7. Brown GC, Magargal LE. The ocular ischaemic syndrome. Clinical, fluorescein angiographic and carotid angiographic features. *Int Ophthalmol* 1988; 11: 239.
8. Jacobs NA, Ridgway AEA. Syndrome of ischaemic ocular inflammation: 6 cases and review. Br J Ophthalmol 1985; 69: 681.
9. Donnan GA, Sharbrough PW, Whisrant JP. Carotid occlusive disease. Effect of bright light on visual evoked response. *Arch Neurol* 1982; 39: 687-9.
10. Sivalingam A, Brown GC, Magargal LE. The ocular ischaemic syndrome. Mortality and systemic morbidity. *Int Ophthalmol* 1989; 13: 187-9.
11. Kawaguchi S, Okuno S, Sakaki T, Nishikawa A. effect of carotid endarteectomy on chronic ocular ischaemic syndrome due to internal carotid artery stenosis. *Neurosurg* 2001; 48(2): 328-32.
12. Kawaguchi S, Sakaki T, Iwahashi H et al. Effect of carotid artery stenting in ocular circulation and chronic ocular ischaemic syndrome. *Cerebrovasc Dis* 2006; 22(5-6): 408.
13. Nagaratnam N, Ghougassian DF, Lewis-Jones M. The shaking limb-a lacunar syndrome. *Postgrad med J* 1988; 64: 311-312.
14. Persoon SL, Kappelle J, Klijn CJM. Limb shaking transient ischaemic attacks in patients with internal carotid occlusion. A case controlled study. *Brain* 2010; 133(3): 915-922.
15. Tatemichi TK, Young WL, Prohovnik I. Perfusion insufficiency in limb shaking transient ischaemic attack. *Stroke* 1990; 21: 341-347.
16. Fisher CM. Lacunar strokes and infarcts: a review. *Neurology* 1982; 32: 871-876.

17. Baquis GD, Passin MS, Scott RM. Limb shaking-a carotid transient ischemic attack *Stroke* 1985; 16: 444-448.

18. Yanagihara T, Piepgras DG, Klass DW. Repetitive involuntary movements associated episodic cerebral ischaemia. *AnnNeurol* 1985; 18: 244-250.

19. Yanagihara T, Klass DW. Rhythmic involuntary movement as a manifestation of transient ischaemic attack. *Am Neurologic Assoc* 1981; 106: 46-48.

20. Ladurner G, Sagez WD, Illef LD, Lechner H. A correlation of clinical findings and CT on ischaemic cerebrovascular disease. *Eur Neurol* 1979; 18: 281-288.

21. Hyland HH, Forman DM. Progress in hemiballismus. *Neurology* 1987; 7: 381-391.

22. Mas JL, Launay M, Deronesne C. Hemiballismus and CT documented lacunar infarct in the lenticular nucleus. *J Neurol Neurosurg Psychiatry* 1987; 50: 104-105.

23. Hertzog C, Schale KW, Gribbin K. Cardiovascular disease and changes in intellectual functioning from middle to old age. *J Gerontol* 1978; 33: 872-883.

24. Poitrenaud J, Vallery-Masson J, Darcet P. et al. Sources of individual differences in cognitive aging: a longitudinal study of an elderly. French managerial population. *Ann Gerontol/Facts and Research in Gerontology* 1994; 8: 462-477.

25. d'Avossa G, Revilla FJ, Grutzendler J. Multi-infarct dementia emedicine,2004. http:www.emedicine.com/NEURO/topic227.htm accessed 4/21/2005.

26. Rao R. The role of carotid stenosis in vascular cognitive impairment. *J Neuro Sci* 2002; 203-204: 103-7.

27. Breteler MMB, Claus JJ, Grobbee DE, Hofman A. Cardiovascular disease distribution of cognitive function in elderly people the Rotterdam study *BMJ* 1994; 308: 1604-1608,

28. Breteler MMB. Atherogenic and hemostatic factors and cognitive function in the elderly. Cognitive decline in the elderly. Rotterdam, Netherlands: Erasmus University. 1993; 74-85. Thesis.

29. Tatemichi TK, Desmond DW, Prohovnikil I, Eidelberg D. Dementia associated with bilateral carotid occlusions: neuropsychological and haemodynamic cause after extracranial to intracranial surgery. *J Neurol Neurosurg Psychiatry* 1995; 58: 633-656.

30. Greiffenstein MF, Brinkman S, Jacob L, Braun P. Neuropsychological improvement following endarterectomy as a function of outcome measure and reconstructed vessel. *Cortex 1988*; 26; 223-230.

31. Grunwald I, Supprian T, Struffert T et al. Cognitive changes after carotid artery stenting. Radiological Society of North American Meeting. (RSNA) November 2005: 350.

32. Pettigrew LC, Thomas N, Howard VJ. et al. Low Mini-Mental Status predicts mortality in asymptomatic carotid arterial stenosis. Asymptomatic Carotid Atherosclerosis Study Investigation. *Neurology* 2000; 55: 30-4.

33. Johnston SC, Oneara ES, Manolio TA. et al. Cognitive impairment and decline are associated with carotid artery disease in patients without clinically evident cerebrovascular disease. *Ann Int Med* 2004; 140: 237-247.

34. Bakker FC, Klijin CJM, Jenneksens-Schinkel A. et al. Cognitive impairment in patients with carotid artery occlusion and ipsilateral transient ishaemic attacks. *J Neurology* 2004; 250: 1340-1347.

35. Ghogawala Z, Westerveld M, Amin-Hanjani S. Cognitive outcomes after carotid revascularization: the role of cereberal emboli and hypoperfusion. *Neurosurgery* 2008; 62: 385-395.

36. Riser M, Gerauld J, Ducondray J et al. Dolico-carotid interne avec syndrome vertiginoux. *Rev Neurol* 1951; 85: 145.

37. Busuttil R, Memsic L, Thomas D. Coiling and kinking of the carotid artery. In Rutherford RB ed Vascular surgery 4th ed. Philadelphia. WB Saunders Company, 1995; 1588-1593.

38. Pellegrino L. Prencipe G. Dolichoartropathies (kinking, coiling tortuousity) of the carotid arteries and atheroscelrotic disease: an ultrasonographic study. *Cardiologia* 1998; 43: 959-966.

39. Weibel J, Fields WS . . . Tortuosity coiling and kinking of the internal carotid artery, relationship of morphological variation to cerebrovascular. *Neurology* 1965; 5: 462-5.

40. Hoskins MS, Scissons RP. Hemodynamically significant carotid disease in duplex ultrasound patients with carotid artery tortuosity. *J Vasc Ultrasound* 2007; 31(1): 11-15.

41. Koskas F, Bahnini A, Walden R, Kieffer E. Stenotic coiling and kinking of the internal carotid artery. *Ann Vasc Surg* 1993; 7: 530-540.

42. Asamoah D, Foy P. Some radiological abnormalities of the cervical carotid artery and their clinical significance. *Clin Radiol* 2009; 30: 93-599.

43. Del Corso L, Moruzzo D, Conte B et al. Tortuosity kinking coiling of the czarotid artery of atherosclerosis or ageing. *Angiology* 1998; 49: 661-71.

44. Milic D, Jovanovic M, Zivic s, Jankovic R. Coiling of the left common carotid artery as a cause of transient ischaemic attack. *J Vasc Surg* 2007; 45(2): 411-413.

45. Koskas F, Bahnini A, Walden R, Kieffer E. Stenotic coiling and kinking of the internal carotid artery. *Ann Vasc Surg* 2005; 7: 530-540.

46. Kraus RR, Bergstein JM, DeBord JR. Diagnosis treatment and outcome of blunt carotid arterial injuries. *Am J Surg* 1999; 178: 190-3.

47. Rajasuriya K, Somasunderam M, Nagaratnam N. Thrombosis of the carotid artery. *Cey Med J* 1960; 4:171-175.

48. Yamaura A, Sukinaga A, Matsumoto T, Maeda Y. Traumatic occlusion of the extracranial internal carotid artery. *The Japan Neurological Society* 1978; 29(12): 1144-1147. [abstract].

49. Hughes PJ. Internal carotid artery occlusion following sports diving. *J R Nav Med Serv* 2000; 80: 120-2

50. Blumrenthal DT, Riggs JE, Oritz O. Carotid artery occlusion following a karate punch to the neck. *Milit Med* 1990; 161: 562-563.

51. Kettaneh AI, Biousse V, Bousser MG. Neurological complications of roller coaster rides: an emerging new risk ? *Presse Med* 2000; 29: 175-180.

52. Singh AK, O'Kudera H, Kobayashi S. Traumatic carotid artety occlusion following blunt cervical injury. *J Clin Neurosci* 1999; 16: 265-268.

13

PRIMARY AND SECONDARY
PREVENTION OF STROKE

Introduction

The risk of first stroke and recurrence of stroke can be reduced by interventions that modify the treatable cardiovascular and cerebrovascular risk factors. Each year it is estimated that there are about 40,000-48,000 stroke events among Australians and about 12,000 suffer a recurrence each year[1]. It is the third greatest single cause of death in Australia. The incidence of stroke increases with age and approximately doubles with each decade after the age of 55 years[2].

Primary and secondary preventive measures are important for the elderly because of the various impacts on the morbidity, mortality and quality of life. The more important risk factors are hypertension, myocardial infarction, atrial fibrillation, diabetes mellitus, dyslipidaemia, and asymptomatic carotid artery stenosis (Table13.1). These risk factors for stroke may be different for the two sexes, ethnic groups and stroke subtypes. Some of the risk factors such as age, gender, race and hereditary factors are non-modifiable. The four life-style factors idendified are cigarette smoking, alcohol consumption, diet and physical inactivity.

Table 13.1 Modifiable risk factors

hypertension

myocardial infarction

atrial fibrillation

diabetes mellitus

dyslipdaemia

asymptomatic carotid artery stenosis

> cigarette smoking
>
> alcohol consumption
>
> physical inactivity

Primary prevention of stroke

A proper understanding of the risk factors is essential for the primary prevention of stroke. Hypertension, congestive heart failure. coronary artery disease and atrial fibrillation are the four major risk factors apart from age for stroke.

Hypertension

The elderly are at high risk for morbidity and mortality from hypertension-related diseases and several studies have shown that treatment of hypertension (isolated systolic hypertension, systolic/diastolic) in the elderly is extremely effective. Hypertension is strongly related to stroke, coronary artery disease (CAD) and renal disease. For every 7.5 mm Hg increase in diastolic blood pressure CAD risk increases by 29% and stroke risk by 46% [3]. It is a modifiable risk factor and its treatment reduces the risk of stroke. There is considerable scientific evidence that treatment with low dose thiazide or thiazide-like diuretics reduces the risk of major cardiovascular events and death in people with hypertension[4]. The Systolic Hypertension in the Elderly Program study (SHEP) showed that treatment of isolated systolic hypertension in the elderly decreased the risk of stroke by 36% [5] and subsequent analysis indicated the greatest benefit may be in those 80 years or older[6]. The European Trial on Isolated Systolic Hypertension in the Elderly[7] was stopped after 2 years because there was a marked decrease in non-fatal and total stroke. Randomized controlled trials of treatment of hypertensive patients 80 years and older revealed by lowering the blood pressure the total mortality could be reduced by one fifth and the rates of cardiovascular events by one-third[8]. Stroke mortality was reduced by 39% in the actively treated patients and all strokes reduced by 30% in the actively treated group. In a trial treatment of 4000 subjects aged 65-74 years with hypertension after 8 years showed a significant reduction of incidence of stroke (25%) and CAD events (19%) in the treated group when compared with the placebo group[9]. The initiation of hypertensive therapy for the 80 years and older are not well defined and should follow the guidelines from the 7th Report of the Joint National Committee[10].

Heart failure (HF) and Coronary Artery Disease (CAD)

After the age of 65 years the incidence of heart failure approximates 10 per 1000 people rising to 100 per 1000 people in those over 80 years[11]. People with heart failure are twice as likely to die from a stroke than the general population. In the community, people with heart failure have an increased risk of ischaemic stroke compared with the general population. Stroke results in more than two-fold increase in mortality[12]. Coronary heart disease, heart failure, dilated cardiomyopathy and heart valve disease have increased risk of stroke.

The presence of heart failure on admission for an acute myocardial infarction increases the in-hospital risk and heart failure treatments may modify the risk of stroke[13]. After myocardial infarction (MI) the incidence of ischaemic stroke approaches 1-2% per year[14]. Studies have demonstrated a reduction in stroke risk with warfarin after MI[15,16]. Antiplatelet agents too have shown to reduce the odds of non-fatal stroke by 39% and non-fatal MI by 31% and vascular death by 15%[17]. Aspirn reduced the relative risk of stroke after MI by approximately 30%. The Scandinavian Simvastatin Survival Study[18] demonstrated a reduction in stroke and transient ischaemic attack in patients with coronary artery disease and higher cholesterol levels.

Atrial Fibrillation

Atrial fibrillation (AF) becomes more prevalent with age in the general population and the extent of stroke associated with AF increases with age[19]. There is a 17-fold increased risk of stroke with rheumatic mitral valve disease with AF. Depending on the type of valve patients with prosthetic valves will require anticoagulation usually with a higher INR.

Non-valvular atrial fibrillation (NVAF) increases the risk of stroke by about 6 times[20,21]. Patients with AF are at increased risk of stroke and patients with NVAF the risk of ischaemic stroke averages 5% per year about 3-5 times that of people in sinus rhythm[20]. Those above 75 years or over or with specific risk factors are highest risk for stroke[22]. AF affects 10% of the elderly over the age of 80 years. The annual risk for stroke increases with increasing age from 11.5% in ages 51-59 to 23% aged 80-89 years[20]. In the United States there are more than 2 million adults with NVAF and about 36% of the strokes were in patients between the ages 80-89 years and was attributed to NVAF [20]. Oral anticoagulation is required in patients with NVAF who have specific risk factors for stroke such as age, previous TIA/stroke, hypertension, diabetes mellitus, heart failure and coronary artery disease. More recently the Atherosclerosis Risk in Communities (ARIIC) study indicated that premature ventricular complexes (PVCs) were associated with new onset of atrial fibrillation and death[23] and an association beteen PVCs and stroke have been reported earlier. PVCs detected on a rhythm strip may be a newly identified marker,[24] if not risk factor for stroke.

CHADS score or CHADS2 score is one method of determining the risk of stroke in patients with AF in primary prevention and as a basis to determine the degree of anticoagulation therapy. The score distinguishes between patients with high risk from low risk of stroke[25,26]. Many clinicians feel that age over 75 years is equally potent risk factor as a history of previous stroke. The European Society of Cardiology (ESC) has recognized this inequality of risk in the CHADS and had put out a more detailed risk assessment tool, the CHA2DS2-VASc score[27] and the CHADS2 score has now been superceded by the former. The CHA2DS2-VASc score has significantly improved the classification of AF patients at low and intermediate risk of stroke[28]. A score of 2 or more is of moderate or high risk and anticoagulation is recommended.

Patients with AF who are on medical prophylaxis are at high risk of bleeding complications and is important to evaluate the risk of bleeding. The European Society of Cardiology in its guidelines released the HAS-BLED score a predictive tool to assess the bleeding risk[29]. The risk factors in the tool includes age 75 years and over, vascular disease and gender. A score of more than 3 indicates high risk[30].

Warfarin is recommended in high risk patients to prevent thromboembolism unless the drug is contraindicated. Warfarin is the more effective although aspirin is most commonly used as an alternative to warfarin. The addition of clopidergrol to aspirin reduces the risk of major vascular events by 11% particularly stroke but increases the risk of major haemorrhage by 57% [31]. According to the ACTIVE-W trial warfarin was more effective than aspirin plus clopidergrol in preventing cerebrovascular events and the danger of bleeding was similar [32].

There is no advantage for patients well controlled on warfarin to switch over to one of the newer anticoagulants. In selected patients an anticoagulant with a direct thrombin inhibition, dabigatran may be an alternative to Vitamin K antagonists like warfarin. Other effective substitutes besides dabigatran for warfarin include factor Xa inhibitors such as apixaban betrixaban and rivaroxaban. Dabigatran has been shown to be equally effective as warfarin in stroke prevention in atrial fibrillation[33]. The RELY study (The Randomised Evaluation of Long-Term Anticoagulation Study) studied patients with nonvalvular AF and at least one risk factor of stroke. Two doses of dabigatran (110mg twice daily or 150 mg twice daily) dose blinded to patients and the researchers weres compared with open-label warfarin with target INR of 2 to 3[32]. The 150 mg twice daily was superior to warfarin in reducing stroke and embolization efficacy with similar risk of bleeding although there was an increase of gastrointestinal bleeding with this dose and seemed to be predominantly in the the age group 75 years and over. The lower dose of 110mg twice daily showed similar efficacy with warfarin in reducing stroke and reduced rates of major bleeding. Both doses however showed a significant reduction of intracranial haemorrhage of about 70% compared with warfarin[33]. Rivaroxaban has also been shown to be effective[34]. The main advantage of dabigatran and rivaroxaban compared to warfarin is that no routine anticoagulation monitoring is required. Furthermore, single dose regimen irrespective of age, gender and body weight should befit most patients. However in case of bleeding there is no antidote available for dabigatran and rivaroxaban. Although the new anticoagulants have an equally effective as warfarin and an equal or better safety profile the choice in selection will become more apparent when they become more widely used.

More recently life threatening haemorrhage have been reported in the elderly with poor renal function taking dabigatran[35,36]. In the old old age group due to age-related decline in the creatinine clearance there is accumulation of dabigatran and hence safe dosing in the elderly will depend on the creatinine clearance. The Cockcroft-Gault formula is the most appropriate method to calculate the creatinine clearance[37].

The aim of treatment of AF is threefold. Firstly the recognition of causal and other associated factors. Secondly the decision as to rate control or correction of the rhythm disturbance and thirdly the prevention of thrombo-embolism. Atrial fibrillation has been classified according to its temporal pattern into first detected episode, paroxysmal, persistent, permanent and recurrent[38].

The first detected AF episode can be paroxysmal or persistent. With the former treatment may not be necessary unless symptomatic but anticoagulation is needed. In the persistent—rate control and anticoagulation or to consider in addition anti-arrhythmic drug therapy and cardioversion.

Chronic AF can be paroxysmal or sustained form (persistent or permanent)[39].

Patients with *paroxysmal* AF have episodes of varying duration and may resolve spontaneously to sinus rhythm. Those with minimal or no symptoms anticoagulation with rate control may suffice. Patients with disabling symptoms besides anticoagulation and rate control, anti-arrhythmic drug therapy and AF ablation if this fails[38].

With *persistent* AF spontaneous conversion is much less likely and conversion to sinus rhythm is either by electrical cardioversion or medications. The former is associated with serious side effects more so in the very elderly. Those with minimal or no symptoms require anticoagulation and rate control. The results of the AFFIRM (atrial fibrillation follow-up investigation of rhythm management) trial[40] revealed that in the elderly population of patients with AF with risk factors for stroke or death rate control is at least as good as rhythm control[41]. In most elderly patients with sustained AF rate control should be a preferred approach[39]. If there are disabling symptoms antiarryhthmic drugs are included and electrical cardioversion as needed. In the elderly the choice of antiarrhythmic drugs is limited. Amiodarone and flecainide are used for medical cardioversion, the latter however is contraindicated with structural heart disease. Other drugs used propafenone and ibutilide. The disadvantages here are the side-effects of the anti-arrhythmic drugs and the recurrence of AF. A new class-3 anti-arrhythmic, dronedrone unlike amiodarone was shown to have no thyroid toxicity and was reported by the ATHENA Investigators[42,43] to reduce the incidence of hospitalization from cardiovascular event but the follow up lasted for only a year.

Patients with *permanent* AF are patients in whom cardioversion has failed or not attempted and cardioversion is not an option to restore sinus rhythm[44]. Management of these patients typically includes anticoagulation and rate control rather than anti-arrhythmic drugs[44]. In patients treated with rate control the medications are used to slow the conduction of the AV node thereby slowing the ventricular rate and the drugs used are a beta-blocker, a calcium channel blocker or digoxin. Beta-blockers are the most effective agents for monotherapy followed by the rate-limiting calcium antagonists like verapamil and diltiazem[45] as these drugs control both exertional and resting heart rate. Digoxin however does not control exertional rate and furthermore the efficacy of digoxin in controlling AF ventricular rate is also limited during paroxysms of AF and is associated with longer attacks[46] and hence it is no longer the drug of first choice for rate control. Continued anticoagulation is mandatory. The disadvantages here are the difficulty to control the rate at times to relieve symptoms and the risks associated with anticoagulation.

Non pharmacological strategies include radiofrequency catheter ablation, use of pacemaker or implantable atrial defibrillator and several surgical treatments. With radiofrequency ablation the success rates are variable and could approximate 75% but this may require multiple procedures especially in patients with permanent AF with higher risk of complications[47]. Patients with paroxysmal AF with structural heart disease and smaller atria are benefitted most with catheter ablation[48]. The MAZE requires cardiac surgery but it is effective in preventing arrhythmia recurrence. Cryomaze procedure using an Argon powered cold probe creates electrical barriers in the upper chamber of the heart blocking the electrical activity permanently. (Table 13.2)

Table 13.2. Treatment of chronic (persistent) Atrial Fibrillation

---

Goals

    rate control

    correction of rhythm

    maintenance of sinus rhythm

        i. Pharmacological to control rate drugs

            beta-blockers

            calcium channel blockers

            digoxin

        to control rhthym

            electrical/medical

        conversion

            followed by anti arrhthymic

        drugs eg amiodarone

            anticoagulation

        ii. Non pharmacological

        in selective patients

        radio frequency catheter ablation

        pacemaker

        implantable atrial defibrillators

Diabetes Mellitus

It is estimated that the risk of stroke increases by 1.5-3 fold for patients with diabetes[49,50,51] and diabetes also doubles the risk of stroke recurrence[52] with poor stroke outcome. Diabetes and stroke together are a major cause of mortality and morbidity worldwide. Many diabetics have hypertension, high cholesterol and increased body weight which increase the stroke risk even more. Diabetic subjects have a very high risk of death from stroke partcularly women[53]. Diabetic subjects without cardiovascular disease have a fatal stroke risk similar to that of non-diabetics with a history of prior stroke and similar risk profile that diabetics may require more aggressive treatment strategies in the future prevention of stroke[54]. In the Collaborative Atovastatin Diabetic Study (CARDS) a randomized trial on type 2 diabetic patients without high LDL cholesterol but with one other risk factor received placebo or atovastatin 10mg daily. Those on Atovastatin treatment showed a significant reduction in the incidence of new stroke by 48% independent of patient's age, gender, cholesterol and blood pressure[55].

Asymptomatic carotid artery stenosis

The risk of stroke among patients with asymptomatic carotid stenosis is relatively low. 45% of stroke patients with asymptomatic carotid stenosis of 60-99% are attributed to lacunes and cardioembolism. These observations could have implications for the use of endarterectomy in asymptomatic patients[56]. The Asymptomatic Carotid Atherosclerosis Surgery (ACAS) trial showed an absolute risk reduction for stroke and death of 5.9% over 5 years with carotid endarterectomy (CE) compared with medical treatment alone in patients with 60%-99% asymptomatic stenosis[57]. The Asymptomatic Carotid Artery Stenosis Trial (ACST) also came up with the almost identical result with 5.4% absolute stroke risk reduction[58]. Several guidelines do not support CE for asymptomatic carotid artery disease. The ACAS and ACST show that elective CE performed by a skilled surgeon is an option when medical management had failed. The American Heart Association guideline however recommends CE for asymptomatic lesions of at least 60% stenosis[59]. Data from randomized controlled studies regarding the efficacy of CE in older patients are limited. NASCET for instance was limited to patients aged < 80 years and only 14% were >75 years. Similarly only 6% of all were >75 years in the ACST. It has been shown recently that there is increasing evidence that the risk of stroke has fallen with best medical treatment alone in patients with severe asymptomatic carotid artery stenosis[60,61]. It is believed that surgery has little to offer except in those patients with a high risk of stroke on medical treatment alone[62].

Dyslipidaemia

Epidemiological studies have indicated a link between total cholesterol levels and ischaemic stroke[63,64]. In a large population study consisting of 17,802 apparently healthy men and women with low levels of low density lipoprotein and increased levels of high sensitivity C-reactive protein using high dose rosuvastatin (20mg per day) the JUPITOR Investigators demonstrated the efficacy of statin for primary prevention of stroke. There were 33 strokes in the rosuvastatin group and almost double the number in the placebo-group[65]. The findings however will need further elucidation and examination. Unlike the association between lipoprotein levels and coronary artery disease no strong correlation between plasma lipoprotein concentrations and risk of stroke has not been clearly established[66]. More recently it has been seen the there is an increased risk of new onset diabetes by 12% with intensive dose statin therapy compared with moderate dose stain therapy[67]. Nevertheless the treatment of dyslipidaemia for the primary dysfunction of ischaemic stroke is based on the recommendations of the National Cholesterol Education Programme (NCEP) Adult Treatment Panel III (ATPIII)[68].

LIFE STYLE FACTORS

i. Cigarrette smoking

Cigarrette smoking has been shown to be an independent determinant of ischaemic stroke[69,70]. It is also an independent determinant of carotid artery plaque thickness[71]. It may increase blood viscosity, increase coagulation, fibrinogen levels., enhance platelet agglutination and raise blood pressure[72]. The risk of stroke increases with the number of cigarettes smoked. Smoking cessation medications and counseling should be offered to all those who smoke.

ii. Alcohol consumption

A J-shaped relationship has been shown between alcohol use—a protective effect in light or moderate drinkers and an elevated stroke risk with heavy alcohol consumption[73]. Alcohol may increase the risk of stroke through various mechanisms that include hypertension, cardiac arrthymias, reduction in cerebral blood flow and hypercoagulable states.

iii. Physical activity

Regular exercise improves functional capacity and reduces the risk of premature stroke from cardiovascular disease. It has been reported as a protective effect on stroke in both men and women[74,75] and that moderate physical activity is more protective against ischaemic stroke than light activity[76]. The ability of exercise training to reduce the mortality and morbidity rates has not been well established for elderly patients. The role of physical activity as a risk factor for stroke is likely mediated through its role in controlling other risk factors such as hypertension, diabetes mellitus and obesity.

iv. Diet

High sodium intake was significant and an independent factor for both cerebral haemorrhage (ICH) and cerebral infarction (CI) in one study[77]. An Australian study reported that additional salt intake increased the risk of ICH but not CI[78].

Sᴇᴄᴏɴᴅᴀʀʏ ᴘʀᴇᴠᴇɴᴛɪᴏɴ ᴏꜰ ꜱᴛʀᴏᴋᴇ

Secondary prevention of stroke includes treatment of hypertension, hyperlipidaemia, antithrombotic therapy for atrial fibrillation, and carotid endarterectomy in patients with severe carotid artery stenosis (Table 13.3).

Table 13. 3 Secondary prevention strategies

Blood pressure reducing agents—hypertension

Lipid lowering agents—hyperlipidaemia

Good glycaemic control-diabetes

Antithrombotic therapy—atrial fibrillation

Anti-platelet agents-myocardial infarction; carotid artery stenosis

Carotid endarterectomy-severe carotid artery stenosis

Attention to lifestyle factors

Hypertension

The perindopril protection against recurrent stroke study (PROGRESS) demonstrated that patients who have had a stroke or TIA on an average 6 months previously and with hypertension when treated with perindopril 4 mg in combination with indapamide 2mg or 2.5 mg at the end of 4 years, the relative risk of stroke was reduced by 28% with similar reduction in all cardiovascvular morbidity. The lowest tertile of mean blood pressure was 128/77mmHg at the point of entry. Patients with intracerebral haermorrhage benefited more than those with ischaemic events[79]. What the trial further showed was that irrespective of the starting blood pressure levels all patients may benefit from treatment to reduce the pressure. The perindopril and indapamide appeared to have been well tolerated as 90% patients continued to take the treatment for 4 years [9].

Another factor is in patients with moderate to severe carotid artery stenosis perindopril may reduce the blood pressure without reducing the global cerebral blood flow. It is now appreciated that TIA and minor stroke have a higher risk of subsequent stroke than before, the 7-day risk is between 8-12% and could be as high as 20% in some groups[80,81]. Whether the benefits of secondary prevention pharmacotherapy extends to the very early period is unclear[82].

Lowering the blood pressure following an acute stroke should be delayed by at least 5-6 days after the onset of the stroke.

Atrial fibrillation (AF)

The recurrence rate is approximately 12% per year for subsequent 2 to 3 years for patients with atrial fibrillation with a history of recent or remote ischaemic stroke.

The more important cardiovascular causes are valvular heart disease, ischaemic heart disease, cardiomyopathies, atrial septal defect, pericarditis, and infiltrative heart diseases such as amyloidosis, endomyocardial fibrosis. The non-cardiovascular causes are hyperthyroidism, pulmonary embolism, idiopathic 'lone' AF, drugs, alcohol, caffeine and pheochromocytoma.

Diabetes

Diabetes is a clear risk factor for stroke[83]. Diabetes and age were independent predictors of recurrent stroke in a population based study of stroke from Rochester, Minn[84] Diabetes doubles the risk of stroke recurrence[51] with poor outcome. Diabetes and stroke together are the major cause of morbidity and mortality worldwide.

Transient ischaemic attack

The American Heart Association and American Stroke Association (AHA/ ASA) in 2008 updated the earlier recommendations for the prevention of stroke in patients with stroke and transient ischaemic attack[85] based on recent trials. They especially looked at two areas requiring modifications namely (i) use of specific antiplatelet agents for stroke prevention in patients with history of noncardioembolic ischaemic stroke or TIA and (ii) use of statins in their prevention of recurrent stroke. Antiplatelet agents rather than oral anticoagulants were recommended for patients with noncardioembolic stroke or TIA. Aspirin (50 to 325mg/d was the new recommendation as monotherapy, the combination of aspirin and extended release of dypramidole and clopidegrol monotherapy as appropriate for initial therapy.

Based on the stroke prevention by Aggressive Reduction in Cholesterol Levels (SPARCL) trial for patients with atherosclerotic ischaemic stroke and TIA and without known coronary heart disease intensive lipid therapy was recommended to reduce risk of stroke and cardiovascular events[86]. Table 13.4 shows the recomendations for the management of secondary prevention of stroke and TIA.

Table 13.4. Recommendations in the management of
secondary prevention of stroke or TIA.

Risk factor	Recommendations
I. Hypertension	Antihypertensive treatment recommended Choice of drugs and targets—according to patient characteristics JNC-7 report- "combination of an ACEI +thiazide type diuretic [10] Lifestyle modifications

II. Hyperlipidaemia

(with CAD or evidence and of atherosclerotic ezetimbe)

Managed according to NCEP III guidelines-lifestyle/diet [87]

NICE strategy [88] statins. Fibrates, nicotinic acid disease, resin who do not tolerate statin. for primary hypercholestraemia

Patients with low HDL cholesterol niacin/ gemfibrozil

III. Carotid artery stenosis

(recurrent TIA
& Ischaemic stroke within last 6 months)

70-90% stenosis CEA *

50-69% CEA recommended depending on patient specific characteristics
(age, gender, comorbidities) below 50% no indication for CEA symptomatic carotid occlusion CEA not recommended
EC/IC

*by surgeon with preoperative mortality or morbidity of <6%
*CEA—carotid endarterectomy

IV. Non-cardiac embolic stroke

Aspirin 50-325 mg/day or dipyramidole or clopidegerol or combined-aspirin
+ dipyramidole. Aspirin
+clopidergrol-increases risk of haemorrhage

V. Atrial fibrillation
VAF

NVAF

anticoagulation unless contraindicated
CHADS score 0—aspirin 325mg/day
CHADS—score   1—aspirin/warfarin
depends on patient preference—INR 2-3
CHADS score 2 or more
-warfarin INR
2-3 [25,26] aged >75 years or over with or without risk factors warfarin

VI. Recent stroke

CT no haemorrhage early anticoagulation with wafarin large infarct risk of haemorrhage aspirin if warfarin is contraindicated if neurological deficits severe consider
QOL with patient/family

Information sources:Gage et al[25]; Gage et al,[26;] NICE[88]; Chobanean et al[10] NCEP,-III[87]

CLINICAL RELEVANCE: Prevention of stroke

* Apart from age, hypertension, coronary artery disease, atrial fibrillation, diabetes, dyslipidaemia and asymptomatic carotid artery stenosis are high risk factors for stroke in the elderly.
* The life style factors include smoking, alcohol consumption, physical inactivity and, diet.
* Those above 75 years or over or with specific risk factors are at highest risk for stroke.
* The initiation of hypertensive therapy for the 80 years and over are not well defined and should follow the guidelines for the 7th Report of the Joint National Committee[10].
* Atrial fibrillation (AF) is increasingly common in the elderly and Non-valvular atrial fibrillation (NAVF) increases the risk of stroke by about 6 times [20,21].
* Oral anticoagulation is required for patients with NVAF who have specific risk factors such as age, previous TIA/stroke, hypertension, diabetes, heart failure and coronary artery disease.
* The decision to prescribe an anticoagulant in the elderly will largely be influenced by such factors as to the presence of co-morbidity, renal function, risk of falls, fraility, concurrent medications such as antiplatelet agents, compliance among others
* There is considerable evidence that the benefit of anticoagulation with warfarin for NVAF in the elderly outweighs the risk of intracerebral haemorrhage in reducing the risk of stroke.
* Warfarin is recommended in high risk patients with AF unless the drug is contraindicated.
* The CHADS2 score is used to determine the risk of stroke patients with AF in primary prevention as well as a basis to determine the degree of anticoagulant therapy.
* The CHA2DS2-VASc is a more embracing risk assessment tool.
* It is meaningful to evaluate the risk of bleeding when anticoagulation is contemplated and the HAS-BLED score is useful to assess the risk of bleeding.
* Patients who are well controlled on warfarin do not benefit by switching over to a new anticoagulant.
* In the prevention of AF related stroke warfarin has been shown to be of proven efficacy, there are however several difficulties in its use for both the clinician and the patient.
* The new anticoagulants, dabigatran, rivaroxaban and apixaban are equally effective and have equal safety profile as warfarin but the decision to prescribe will become more apparent only with their wider use.

* Dabigatran is easier to use and equally effective and no routine monitoring is required and safe dosing in the elderly will depend on the creatinine clearance.

* Antiplatelet agents rather than oral anticoagulants are recommended for patients with noncardioembolic stroke or TIA.

* In the elderly patient with AF with risk factors for stroke and rate control with anticoagulation is as good as rhythm control[41].

* In patients with permanent (chronic) AF electrical cardioversion is associated with serious side effects especially in the elderly and is not an option to restore sinus rhythm.

* There should be regular review, continued and strict monitoring of all elderly who are on oral anticoagulants.

* Patients aged 80 years or more with TIA or ischaemic stroke have been under investigated and the screening for carotid artery disease in symptomatic patients is singularly meaningful and evidence of considerable benefit from endarterectomy.

* Patients 80 years or more should not be excluded from carotid endarterctomy solely on age.

* The efficiency of statin in primary prevention has recently been demonstrated[86].

REFERENCES

1. Australian Institute of Health and Welfare (AIHW). Incidence and prevalence of chronic diseases. *http://www.aihw.gov.au/c/darf/data_pages/incidence_prevalence.*
2. Wolf PA. Risk factors for stroke. *Stroke.* 1985; 16(3): 359-360.
3. Reynolds E, Baron RB. Hypertension in women and the elderly. *Postgrad Med* 1996; 100:
4. Pstay BM, Lumley T, Furberg CD et al. Health outcomes associated with various antihypertensive therapies used as first line agents: a network meta-analysis *JAMA* 2003; 289: 2534-44.
5. SHEP. Co-operative Research Group-Prevention of stroke by antihypertensive drug treatment in older persons with isolated systolic hypertension. Final results of the Systolic Hypertension in Elderly Program (SHEP). *JAMA* 1991; 265: 3255-60.
6. SHEP. The Systolic Hypertension in the Elderly Program (SHEP). Cooperative Research Group. Implications of the Systolic Hypertensionin the Elderly Program. *Hypertension.* 1993; 21: 335-343.
7. Staessen JA, Fagard R, Thijis L. et al. Morbidity and mortality in placebo-controlled European Trial on Isolated Systolic Hypertension in the elderly. *Lancet* 1997; 350: 757-764.
8. Susman ER. Treatment of high blood pressure appears worthwhile in very elderly patients. Presented at AIC *http://www.docguide.com/news/content.nsf/news852571020057CCF6852574210060264.*
9. MRC Working Party. Medical Research Council trial of treatment of hypertension in older adults: preliminary results. *Br Med J* 1992; 304: 405-12.
10. Chobanian AV, Bakrus JA, Black HR et al. The Seventh report of the Joint National Committee on prevention detection, evalualtion and treatment of high blood pressure. The JNC Report *JAMA* 2003; 289: 2560-7.
11. Sharpe N. Heart failure in the community. *Prog Cardiovasc Dis.* 1998; 41: 73-76.
12. Witt BJ, Brown RD, Jacobsen ST et al. Ischaemic stroke after heart failure: community study. *Am Heart J 2006*; 152(1): 102-9.
13. Szummer KE, Solomon SD, Velazquez EJ et al. Heart failure on admission and the risk of stroke following acute myocardial infarction: the VALIANT registry. *Eur Heart J* 2005; 26(20): 2116-2119.
14. 4th American College of Chest Physicians Consensus Conference on Antithrombotic Therapy. Tuscon, Arizona. April 1995. Proceedings *Chest* 1995; 108 (suppl 4): 2255-5225.
15. Smith P, Arnesen H, Holme I. The effect of warfarin on mortality and reinfarction after myocardial infarction. *N Engl J Med* 1990; 323: 147-152.

16. Anticoagulants in Secondary Prevention of Events in Coronary Thrombosis (ASPECT). Research Group. Effect of long-term oral anticoagulant treatment on mortality and cardiovascular morbidity after myocardial infarction. *Lancet* 1974; 343: 499-503.

17. Antiplatelets Trialists Collaboration. Collaborative overview of randomised trials of antiplatelet therapy: Prevention of death, myocardial infarction and stroke by prolonged antiplatelet therapy in various categories of patients. *BMJ* 1994; 308: 81-106.

18. Randomised trial of cholesterol lowering in 4444 patients with coronary heart disease: the Scandinavian Simvastatin Survival Study. *Lancet* 1994; 344: 1383-89.

19. Marini C, De Santos F, Sacco S et al. Contribution of atrial fibrillation to incidence and outcome of ischaemic stroke results from a population based study. *Stroke* 2005; 30: 1115-1119.

20. Wolf PA, Abbott RD, Kannel WD Atrial fibrillation as an independent risk factor for stroke: the Framingham Study. *Stroke* 1991; 22: 983-988.

21. Wolf PA, Dawbr TAR, Thomas HEJ et al. Epidemiologic assessment of chronic atrial fibrillation and risk of stroke: the Framingham Study. *Neurology* 1978; 28: 973-977.

22. Singer DF. Anticoagulation to prevent stroke in atrial fibrillation and its implications for managed care. *Am J Cardiol* 1998; 81: 850-

23. Agarwal SK, Heiss G, Rautaharju PM et al. Premature ventricular complexes and risk of incident stroke: the Atherosclerosis Risk in Communities (ARIC) Study. *Stroke* 2010; 41: 588-593.

24. Worthington JM, Gattellari M, Leung DY. 'Where There's Smoke . . ." Are premature ventricular complexes a new risk factor for stroke?. *Stroke* 2010; 41: 572-573.

25. Gage BF, van Walraven C, Pearce L et al. Selecting patients with AF for anticoagulation: stroke risk stratification in patients taking aspirin. *Circulation* 2004; 110: 2287-92.

26. Gage BF, Waterman AD, Shannon W et al. Validation of clinical classification schemes for predicting stroke results from the National Registry of Atrial fibrillation. *JAMA* 2001; 285: 2860-70.

27. Lip GYH, Frison L, Halperin JL, Lane DA. Identifying patients at high risk stratification schemes in an anticoagulated atrial fibrillation cohort. Stroke 2010;41: 2731-2738 (abstract).

28. Olesen JB, Torp-Pedersen C, Hansen ML, Lip GY. The value of score for refining stroke risk.stratification in patients with atrial fibrillation with a CHADS2 score 0-1: a nationwide cohort study. *Thromb Haemost* 2012;197(6): 1172-9(abstract).

29. European Heart Rhythm Association; European Association for cardio-Thoracic Surgery, Camm AJ, Kirchhof P, Lip GY, Schotten U, et al. Guidelines for the management of atrial fibrillation: The task Force for the Management of

Atrial Fibrillation of the European Society of Cardiology (ESC) *Eur Heart J* 2010;31:2369-429.

30. Lip GY. Implications of CHA2DS2-VASc and HAS-BLED scores for thromboprophylaxis in atrial fibrillation. *Am J Med* 2011;124(2):111-4 (abstract).

31. Connolly SJ, PogueJ, Hart RG et al. ACTIVE Invesyigators. Effect of clopidergrol added to aspirin in patients with atrial fibrillation. *N Eng J Med* 2009;360:2066-78.

32. Connolly S, Pogue J, Hart R et al. ACTIVE investigators. Clopidergrol plus aspirin versus oral anticoagulation for atrial fibrillation in the Atrial Fibrillation Clopidergrol Trial with Irbesartan for the prevention of Vascular EVENTS (ACTIVE W): a randomized controlled trial. *Lancet* 2006;367:1903-12.

33. Connolly S, Ezekowitz MD, Yusuf S et al. Dabigatran vs warfarin in patients with atrial fibrillation. *NEJM* 2009;361:1139-1151.

34. Galllus A. New oral anticoagulants-clinical applications. Aust Presccr 2010;33:42-47.

35. Legrand M, Mateo L, Ariband A et al. The use of dabigatran in elderly patients. *Arch Intern Med* 2011;171:1281-1286.

36. Harper P, Young PL, Merriman L. Bleeding risk with dabigatran in the frail elderly. *N Eng J Med* 2012;366:864-865.

37. Meliom C, Peterson ED, Chen AV et al. Cockcroft-Gault versus modification of diet in renal disease: importance of glomerular filtration rate formula for classification of chronic kidney disease in patients with non-ST segment elevation acute coronary syndrome. *J Am Coll Cardiol* 2008;51:991-996.

38. Fuster V, Ryden LE, Asinger RW et al. ACC/AHAESC guidelines for the management of patients with atrial fibrillation executive summary a report of the American College of Cardiology/American Heart Association task force in practice guidelines and the European Society of Cardiology committee for practice guidelines and policy conferences (committee to develop guidelines for the management of patients with atrial fibrillation developedin collaboration with the North American Society of Pacing and Electrophysiology. *Circulation* 2001;101:2118-50.

39. Lip GYH, Li Saw Hee FL. Paroxysmal atrial fibrillation.*QJM* 2001;94(12):665-678.doi:10.1093/qjmed/94.12.665.

40. Wyse DG, Waldon AL, DiMarco JP. et al. A comparison of rate control and rhythm control in patients with atrial fibrillation. *N Engl J Med* 2002;347:1825-33.

41. Markides V, Schilling RJ. Atrial fibrillation: classification, pathophysiology, mecahnisms and drug treatment. *Heart* 2003;89:939-942.

42. Connolly SJ, Crijns HJ, Torp-Pedersen C, et al. for the ATHENA investigators. Analysis of stroke in ATHENA: a placebo-controlled double-blind, parallel-arm trial to assess the efficacy of dronedarone: 400 mg BID for the prevention of

cardiovascular hospitalization or death from any cause in patients with atrial fibrillation/atrial flutter. *Circulation* 2009; 120:1174-1180.

43. Hohnloser SH, Crijns HJGM, van Eickels M.et al. for the ATHENA Investigators. Effect of dronedarone on cardiovascular events in atrial fibrillation. *N Engl J Med* 2009; 360: 668-678.

44. Fuster V, Ryden LE, Cannom DS et al. ACC/AHA/ESC 2006 Guidelines for the management of paients with atrial fibrillation. *Eur Heart J* 2006;27:1979-2030.

45. Olshansky B, Rosenfeld LE, Warner AL. et al. The atrial fibrillation follow-up investigation of rhythm management (AFFIRM) study: approaches to control rate in atrial fibrillation. *J Am Coll Cardiol* 2004; 43: 1201-1208.

46. Rawles JM, Metcalfe MJ, Jennings K. Time of occurrence, duration and ventricular rate of paroxysmal atrial fibrillation: the effects of digoxin. *Br Heart J.* 1990;63: 225-7 (abstract).

47. Pappone C, Santinelli V. Ablation of atrial fibrillation. Eur Cardiovasc Dis 2008;4:96-98.

48. Kalman JM, Sanders P, Brieger DB et al. National Heart Foudation of Australia consensus statement on catheter ablation as a therapy for atrial fibrillation. MJA 2013;198:27-28.

49. Stegmayr B, Asplund K, Diabetes as a risk factor for stroke. A population perspective. *Diabetologia.*1995; 30:736-43.

50. Stamler J, Vaccaro PO, Neaton JD et al. Diabetes, other risk factors and 12 cardiovascular mortality for screened in the Multiple Risk Factor Intervention Trial. Diabetes. *Diabetes Care* 1993, 16: 434-44

51. Kisela BM, Khoury J, Kleindorfer D. et al. Epidemiology of ischaemic stroke in patients with diabetes: the greater Cincinnati? Northern Kentucky Stroke Study. *Diabetes Care* 2005; 28: 355-9

52. Hankey GJ, Jamrozik K, Broadhurst RJ et al. Long term risk of first recurrent stroke in the Perth Community Stroke Study. *Stroke* 1998; 29: 2491-500.

53. Tuomilehto J, Rastenyte D, Jousilahti P et al. Diabetes mellitus as a risk factor for death from stroke. *Stroke* 1996; 27: 210-215.

54. Ho JE, Paultre F Mosca L Is diabetes mellitus and cardiovascular disease risk equivalent for fatal stroke in women? *Stroke* 2003; 34: 2812.

55. Colhoun HM, Betteridge DJ, Durrington PM et al. CARDS. Investigations. Primary prevention of cardiovascular disease with atorvastatin in type 2 patients in the Collaborative Atovarstatin Diabetes Study (CARDS): multicentre randomized placebo-controlled trial. *Lancet.* 2004; 304: 685-96.

56. Inzitari D, Elaszin M, Gates P et al. The causes and risk of stroke in patients with asymptomatic carotid artery stenosis. *New Eng J Med.* 2000; 342: 1693-1701.

57. The executive committee for the Asymptomatic Carotid Atherosclerosis Study Endarterectomy for asymptomatic carotid artery stenosis. *JAMA* 1995; 273: 1421-8.

58. MRC Asymptomatic Carotid Surgery Trial (ACST) Collaborative Group. Prevention of disabling and fatal strokes by successful carotid endarterectomy in patients without neurological symptoms: randomized controlled trial. *Lancet* 2004; 363: 1491-502,

59. Biller J, Feinberg WM, Castaldo JF et al. Guidelines for carotid endarterectomy: a statement for health care professionals from a Special Writing of Stroke Council, American Heart Association. *Circulation* 1998; 97: 501-09.

60. Abbott AL. Medical (nonsurgical) intervention alone is now the best treatment for the prevention of stroke associated with asymptomatic severe carotid stenosis: results of a systemic revierw and analysis. *Stroke* 2009; 40: e573-e583.

61. Marquardt L, Geraghty OC, Mehta Z et al. Low risk of ipsilateral stroke in patients with asymptomatic carotid stenosis on best medical treatment: prospective population based study. *Stroke* 2009; 2010; 41.

62. Goldstein LB, Rothwell PM. Advances in prevention and health services delivery 2009. *Stroke* 2010; 41: e71-e73.

63. Zhang X, Patel A, Haribe H et al. Cholesterol, coronary heart disease and stroke in the Asia Pacific region. *Int J Epidemiol* 2006;32(4):563-72.

64. Kurth T, Everett BM, Buring JE et al. Lipid levels and the risk of ischaemic stroke in women. Neurology 2007;68(8):556-62.

65. Ridker PM, Daneilson ED, Fonseca FAH et al. for the JUPITOR Study Group. Rosuvastatin to prevent vascular events in men and women with elevated C-reactive protein. *N Engl J Med* 2008; 359: 2195-2207.

66. Fine-Edelstein JS, Wolf PA, O'Leary DH et al. Precursors of extracranial carotid atherosclerosis in the Framingham Study. *Neurology* 1994; 44(6):1046-1050.

67. Preiss D, Seshasai SR, Welsh P. et al. Risk of incident diabetres with intensive-dose compared with moderate dose statin therapy" a meta-analysis. *JAMA.* 2011;305:2556-64.

68. Grundy SM, Cleeman JI, Merz CN. et al, Implications of recent clinical trials for the National Cholesterol Education Programme Adult treatment Panel III guidelines. *Circulation* 2004;110(2): 227-9.

69. Abbott RD, Yin Y, Reed OM et al. Risk of stroke in male cigarette smokers. *N Engl J Med.*1986; 315: 717-720.

70. Gorelick PB, Rodin MB, Langerbeig P et al. Weekly alcohol consumption, cigarette smoking and risk of ischaemic stroke: reults of a case-control study at 3 uran medical centers in Chicago Illnios. *Neurology* 1989;39:339-343.

71. Sacco RL, Roberts JK, Boden-Albala R et al. For The Northern Manhattan Stroke Study: Race-ethnicity and determinants of carotid atherosclerosis in a multiethnic population. *Stroke* 1987; 28: 929-935.

72. Wolf PA. Cigarettes, alcohol and stroke *N Engl J Med.* 1986; 315: 1087-89.

73. Gill JS, Zezulka AV, Shipley MI et al. Stroke and alcohol consumption. *N Engl J Med.* 1981; 315: 1041-1046.

74. Kiely DK, Wolf PA, Cupples LA et al. Physical activity and stroke risk. The Framingham Study. *Am J Epidemiol* 1994; 140: 608-620.

75. Manson JE, Stampfer MJ, Willett WC. Physical activity and incidence of coronary heart disease and stroke in women. *Circulation.* 1995; 91: 927.

76. Sacco RL, Boden-Albala B, Gu Q et al. Any physical activity reduces ischaemic stroke risk. The Northern Manhattan Stroke Study. *Neurology* 1996; 40: 400.

77. Choi-Kwan S, Kim JS. Lifestyle factors and risk of stroke in Seoul, South Korea. *J Stroke Cerebrovasc Dis* 1998;7: 414-420.

78. Jamrozik K, Broadhurst RJ, Anderson CS et al. The role of lifestyle factors in the etiology of stroke: A population based case-control study in Perth. Western Australia. *Stroke* 1994; 25: 51-59.

79. Randomised trial of perindopril based blood pressure lowering regimen among 6,105 individuals with previous stroke or transient ischaemic attack. Lancet 2001;358:1033-1034.

80. Johnston SC, Gress DR, Browner WS, Sidney S. Short-term prognosis after emergency department diagnosis of TIA. *JAMA* 2000: 284: 2901-6

81. Coul AJ, Lovett JK, Rothwell PM. A population based study of the early risk of stroke after a transient ischaemic or minor stroke: implications for public education and organization services. *BMJ* 2004; 328: 326-8.

82. Muir KW. Secondary prevention for stroke and transient ischaemic attacks Editorial. *BMJ* 2004; 328: 297-98.

83. Kannel WB, McGee DL. Diabetes and cardiovascular disease. The Framingham study *JAMA.*1979; 241: 2035-2038.

84. Petty GW, Brown RD Jr, Whisnant JP. et al. Survival and recurrence after first central infarction: a population based study in Rochester. Minnesota 1975 through 1989. *Neurology* 1998; 50: 208-216.

85. Adams RJ, Albers G, Albert MJ et al. Update to the AHA/ASA Recommendations for the Prevention of Stroke in Patients With Stroke and Transient Ischaemic Attack. *Stroke* 2008;39:1647-1652

86. Amarenco P, Bogousslavsky J, Callihan A.3rd. et al. Stroke Prevention by Aggressive Reduction in Cholesterol Levels (SPARCL). Investigations. High dose artovastatin after stroke or transient ischaemic attack. *N Engl J Med* 2006;355:549-559.

87. The Third Report of the National Cholesterol Evaluation Program (NCEP). www:nhlbi.nih.gov/guidelines/cholesterol/atp3fall.pdf

88. NICE (May 2008). Lipid modification—cardiovascular risk association and the modification of blood lipids for the primary and secondary prevention of cardiovascular disease.

14

NEUROPSYCHIATRIC DISORDERS

POSTSTROKE

Introduction

Neuropsychiatric disorders following stroke are common and serious. The most frequent poststroke psychiatric syndrome is depression. Mania, anxiety and psychotic disorders occur after cerebrovascular disorders.

Pathophysiology

Primary depressive disorder has been divided into 'early onset' and 'late onset' (LOD) disorders. The late—onset is closely linked to clinical and neuroimaging evidence of cerebrovascular disease[1,2] and there is a growing awareness of the influence of vascular based LOD and 'late onset mania'(LOM) lending support to distinct vascular subtypes. The 'vascular hypothesis' is upheld by comorbidity of depression, vascular risk factors, vascular disease and the association with ischaemic lesions to characteristic behavioural symptoms[3]. In a study to compare the frequency of depression, 670 geriatric rehabilitation patients were grouped into those with no evidence of vascular disease, those with cerebrovascular risk factors but no stroke and those with stroke only[4]. The study revealed the frequency of depression in patients without stroke increased as cerebrovascular risk factors increased. Hence the term 'vascular depression' is often used to described this syndrome[5]. Cerebral infarction, including silent infarction, transient ischaemic attack and small vessel disease or white matter hyperintense lesions on magnetic resonance imaging can cause characteristic vascular syndromes.

Functional excess of several neurotransmitters including serotonin, dopamine and noradrenaline can give rise to affective disorder rather than the direct anatomical damage caused by the lesions. It may be asked how similar neuroanatomical changes can give rise to syndromes whose features are not uniform. According to Cummings[6] the occurrence of different psychological syndromes can be influenced by several factors such as genetic constitution, age of onset, personality characteristics, early life experiences and exact location and extent of the lesion among others.

I. Post-stroke depression
Introduction

Post stroke depression (PSD) is a serious disorder following stroke but is often overlooked and left untreated[7]. Poststroke depression has been underdiagnosed in 50-80% of cases by nonpsychiatric physicians[8]. Compared to age-matched controls stroke survivors have a 6-fold risk of developing clinically overt depression even after more than 2 years following the initial insult[9]. Patients with a history of psychiatric disorder have been found to have high rate of PSD[10]. Depression can occur months to years after the stroke[11,12]. PSD may involve a spectrum of mood disorders, major and minor depression, vascular depression and dementia—related depression[13]. It inhibits recovery and limits quality of life[14]. Regardless of the lesion location depression is common in delayed stroke recovery[15] for PSD patients are less likely to participate in their rehabilitation[16].

Incidence prevalence and epidemiology

The most frequent psychiatric syndrome after stroke is depression (PSD). Approximately 20% of the patients who sustained a stroke met the criteria for major depression post-stroke and 20% the criteria for minor depression[17]. The frequency of PSD has been estimated between 10-60% [18] depending on the diagnostic criteria used, time lapse after onset of stroke and selection of patients. Pooled data revealed the prevalence rates for major depression to be 19.3% among hospitalized patients and 23.5% among outpatient samples [19]. The frequency and severity of depression increased significantly during the period six months to two years after stroke[20]. Mortality in PSD is estimated between 3.5 and 10 times higher than in non—depressed stroke patients and suicide ideation occurred in 11.8% of stroke patients[18]. Poststroke depression is more common in women than in men.

Pathophysiology

Major depression is said to be significantly more frequent with left anterior lesions (frontal or basal ganglia) whereas minor depression occurs with either right or left occipital lesions[21] but has not been demonstrated in further epidemiological studies[20]. Recent studies have revealed that left anterior cerebral or subcortical lesions may lead to development of major depression and that pre-existing subcortical atrophy may play an important role[21]. Severe affective depression was associated with left frontal lobe lesions whereas apathetic depression was mostly involved the basal ganglia[23]. In a recent study Santos et al[24] reported that it is the amassed vascular affliction resulting from chronic accumulation of lacunal infarcts within the thalamus, basal ganglia and deep white matter which may be more important than single infarcts in the prediction of PSD. Other studies have found that lesion location does not play an important role in depression after stroke[25,26].

PET scan findings have shown a difference in the biochemical response in the two hemispheres to stroke. The serotonin receptor binding is increased in the right hemisphere compared to the left suggesting that lower the serotonin binding the more severe the depression[22]. Several factors increase the likelihood of PSD-localisation and severity of the brain lesion, reduction in serotonin and dopamine and other transmitter levels, premorbid personality, patient's age and social isolation[27,28] and possibly a family history of major depression[17]. For several years increase in the synaptic concentrations of serotonin, noradrenaline and/or dopamine were the basis for pathophysiological models of depression[29]. More lately there has been considerable move towards embodying structural brain changes in frontal, subcortical and medial temporal structures[30-32].

Diagnosis

Vascular depression predating stroke is associated with psychomotor retardation, older age of onset, greater degree of cognitive impairment and less feeling of guilt than seen in major depression[3,33]. Screening for depression should be part of all patients undergoing stroke rehabilitation. The diagnosis is hard for it may be difficult to distinguish which symptoms are due to the stroke and which are due to depression. It is difficult to establish the diagnosis in stroke patients especially in patients with cognitive impairment, aphasia and anosognosia. These may hinder interview-based diagnostic approaches. At present poststroke depression should be based on mental state examination and DSM-IV criteria for depression due to stroke[19].

Treatment

Early diagnosis and treatment of PSD is crucial. Treatment principles are broadly similar to those currently used to treat non-organically ill patients[34]. Treatment of post stroke depression requires not only the need to actively manage the stroke condition but also active and appropriate use of other behavior and psychological therapy[29]. In the older patient the first line of treatment are the SSRIs or venlafaxine and if there is no reponse or partial response mirtazapine or bupropion can be used. The third line of treatment is the use nortriptyline or despiramine if there is partial or no response to the former medications.

Selective serotonin reuptake inhibitors (SSRIs) may be the first line treatment of poststroke depression. They have few side effects, low toxicity and moderate efficacy[29]. The SSRIs and their main adverse effects include, sertraline (agitation, tremor, dizziness and decreased libido), fluoxetine (agitation,), paroxetine (insomnia), citalopram (sexual dysfunction and anticholinergic effects) and escitalopram (similar to citalopram). The bicyclic (SNRI) venlafaxine causes cardiovascular and discontinuation effects and the nor-epinephrine and dopamine-reuptake inhibitor bubropion, agitation, lowers seizure threshold and insomnia and serotonin antagonist,

179

mirtazapine sedation and weight gain. Although tricylclic depressants (TCAs) have increased side effects and are highly toxic in a double-blind study nortriptyline was found to be both well tolerated and superior to fluoxetine in the treatment of poststroke depression[35] and should be strongly considered for treating poststroke depression[17]. The secondary amines tricyclics cause cardiovascular and anicholinergic effects. The tricyclics should be taken at bedtime.

II MANIA

Introduction

The term 'manic syndrome' in old age has its critics because of the high occurrence of medical and neurological conditions in old people with overall incidence of late—onset mania. Several neurological conditions have been correlated with secondary mania.

Incidence prevalence and epidemiology

There were only three cases of post-stroke mania among 700 stroke patients studied[36]. Fujikawa et al[37] studied the incidence of silent cerebral infarction (SCI) in patients with major depression and found half the cases of late-onset mania to be secondary mania related to SCI and often associated with large areas of brain damage as compared with late—onset depression.

Pathophysiology

With secondary mania the strongest association is with lesions in the right hemisphere which has connections with the frontal lobes[38]. There are also a growing number of reports of secondary mania following left hemispheric stroke[39-43] and the lesions are in the fronto-temporal, frontal, temporal and basal ganglia regions[41]. The lesions in secondary mania following stroke are also seen in the limbic or limbic-connected areas, orbito-frontal[44,45], basotemporal,[45] head of caudate and thalamus[46], and ventral pontine infarction involving the left or right side[47].

It is also well known that the left medial thalamus and paramedian territory[48,49] and left polar thalamic regions[50] are massively connected to the frontal structures and that their damage may result in frontal lobe dysfunction. Two patients with secondary mania frontal lobe dysfunction and dementia syndrome following right posterior cerebral artery territory infarction have been reported[51-52] with likely involvement of the frontal-subcortical circuitry and frontal diencephalic brain stem system.

Alexander et al [53] proposed five segregated circuits and each circuit linked the striatum, globus pallidus, sunbstantia and the thalamus with topographically organized divisions of the frontal cortex. Involvement of the orbitofrontal circuit gives rise to tactlessness, disinhibition and impulsivity. Secondary mania occurs with lesions affecting the orbitofrontal-subcortical circuit[54,55]. Several transmitters and modulators are involved in the fronto-subcortical circuits.

Discussion

Diagnosis is by fulfilment of DSM-IV criteria for mania by clinical review. This broadly includes elevated mood, flight of ideas, rapid pressured speech, impaired judgment, and decreased sleep among others. The diagnosis of secondary mania is the satisfaction of the criteria of Krauthammer and Klerman[56] namely, the presence of elevated or irritable mood together with at least two of the symptoms in the diagnosis of mania, symptoms duration of at least one week and no history of affective disorder and confusion.

Establishing a causal relationship between manic symptoms and specific medical condition can be difficult as to whether it is the cause or merely a precipitant. Neurological lesions are commonly associated with symptoms that may be diagnosed or labelled as psychiatric.

Treatment

Case reports have suggested that lithium, valproic acid, carbamazepine, clonidine and neuroleptics may each be effective in the treatment of poststroke mania. It has been suggested that mood stabilizing anticonvulsants may be the agents of choice in the treatment of secondary mania and given the propensity for seizures in the poststroke period[17]. Generally, patients respond to neuroleptics but in some treatment resistant cases anticonvulsants are useful [57]. Open trials in the elderly and other groups with secondary mania has shown divalproex sodium to be effective and well tolerated[58].

III. ANXIETY DISORDERS

Introduction

Anxiety symptoms can be primary or secondary to other physical or psychiatric disorders. It often occurs with post stroke depression (PSD). Several studies have supported the existence of significant co-morbidity between poststroke anxiety and PSD[59]. Comorbidity with major depression seemed to impair the prognosis of depression[60].

Incidence prevalence and epidemiology

Anxiety disorder was found in 26% in men and 36% in women following stroke respectively[61]. In a study of 288 stroke patients 27% met the DSM-III criteria for generalized anxiety disorder[62]. In a 3-year longitudinal study of 80 patients with acute stroke the prevalence of GAD showed no reduction from the acute stage (28%) and major depression was seen in 85% of poststroke GAD patients at some stage during the 3-year period [60]. House et al [63] reported a prevalence of 3% for agoraphobia and 1% for GAD 6 months after stroke from Oxfordshire Community Stroke Project.

181

Pathophysiology

It has been reported that anxiety alone was associated with left hemispheric lesions and depression and anxiety with left cortical lesions[62]. At 3-years after the stroke GAD was significantly associated with both cortical and subcortical atrophy[60]. There are reports of less common emotional disorders such as panic attacks with social phobia following a focal lesion in the temporal lobe[64] and obsessive-compulsive disorders in vascular lesions of the caudate and globus pallidus[65].

Many believe that the role of neurotransmitters in the experience of anxiety is complex. Evidence suggests that GAD involves several neurotransmitter systems in the brain including norepinephrine and serotonin. Other studies have shown that the receptors in the brain for GABA are blocked.

Diagnosis

Astrom[60] found difficulty in diagnosis of anxiety disorders in medically ill patients, especially that of panic disorder, phobic behaviour, agoraphobia and social phobia but concluded that they had significant negative impact on psychosocal life and relationships. Apart from decreased energy all other symptoms of GAD are significantly more frequent among patients with anxiety[66]. Poststroke GAD can be diagnosed by using the DSM-IV symptom criteria[14].

Treatment

There are no systematic treatment studies of poststroke GAD and only data available is from treatment of GAD without stroke. Benzodiazapines should be used with caution in older people. Buspirone has similar efficacy to diazepam but a more acceptable side-effects profile [67]. The most well studied treatment is cognitive behavioural therapy (CBT).

IV. Post stroke psychosis

Psychotic symptoms of delusions and hallucinations are rarely described in stroke patients [68,69].

Incidence and prevalence

Delirious ideation was seen in 15 of 360 patients with acute stroke within 24 hours of onset[70]. Rabins et al [68] studied stroke patients more than 60 years over a 9-year period (n=1191) and identified only 5 with psychosis.

Pathophysiology

Psychosis has been generally reported with right hemispheric stroke[71] especially tempero-parieto-occipital regions[68, 69] or the thalamus[72]. Right parietal lesions, subcortical atrophy and seizures may be risk factors for developing psychosis after stroke[58]. Manic delirium has been reported as the main symptom of right—sided thalamic infarct with SPECT findings suggesting a frontal or limbic connection as the cause[72].

Diagnosis

The psychiatric symptoms include delusions and hallucinations which may involve various sensory modalities such as auditory and visual hallucinations, ideas of reference and regressed motor behaviour[13]. Distinguishing poststroke psychosis with delusions and hallucinations from PSD and poststroke dementia can be difficult A history of premorbid psychiatric illness can be helpful[13].

Treatment

Generally patients respond to neuroleptic medications. Treatment includes atypical antipsychotics such as risperidone 0.5 to 1mg po or olanzapine 2.5 mg po. In those resistant anticonvulsants have been useful[69]. Although very rarely minor strokes have been reported with these medications their clinical significance appears small[13].

DELUSIONAL DISORDERS

Introduction

A number of neuropsychiatric disturbances have been described following stroke including delusional disorders. The older the patient the more likely are delusions to be organic than functional. i. Delusions concerning infidelity of the spouse (Orthello syndrome) can be one of a number of manifestations of paranoid psychosis or it may occur as a monosymptomatic delusional belief[6]. Delusional jealousy occurs in organic psychosis, paranoid disorders, alcohol psychosis, schizophrenia and to a lesser extent affective disorder[73].

Incidence prevalence epidemiology

The occurrence of delusional jealousy in the elderly psychiatric population is 1.4%[74].

Pathophysiology

It has been described following a right middle artery infarct[75], in the acute phase of cerebellar infarction associated with distortion of the brain stem[76], and pontine infarction where the patient's mood was associated with a mixture of anger, irritability, apprehension and occasionally to physical violence[77]. Post stroke psychiatric disorders might be a consequence of structural damage to neuronal pathways or to abnormalities of some of the brain's chemical transmitter systems. Lesions in a variety of locations could give rise to delusions[75] when the lesions disrupts the ascending monoaminogenic projections from the brain stem to the cortex via the basal ganglia and adjacent structures[6].

Diagnosis

The Othello syndrome could present with hostility ranging from verbal threats to homicidal acts and could have serious impact on domestic and public safety[78]. Patients are firmly convinced of the infidelity of the spouse in spite of contrary evidence.

Treatment

Delusional disorders are often treated with atypical antipsychotics—risperidone, quetiapine and olanzapine. Cognitive therapy has shown promise. Pharmacotherapy can be combined with cognitive therapy with benefit.

ii. Delusional parasitosis is a belief that the skin is infested with worms, insects or organisms. It could be produced by a variety of organic processes: toxic, metabolic and by structural disorders (secondary delusional parasitosis).

Incidence prevalence epidemiology

Annual prevalence of delusional parasitosis is estimated at 80 per million people with a yearly incidence of 20 per million[79]. Heim and Mogner [81]described a prevalence of 9% of delusional infestation.

Pathophysiology

Delusional parasitosis and organic delusional disorders share a common topography of brain lesions involving subcortical and limbic brain areas and have been associated with lesions in either hemispheres[81], and with lesions in various sites for instance, the right temporo-parietal—occipital[82], left temporo-parietal[83], right basal ganglia and occipito-temporal cerebral infarctions[84]. It is hypothesised that delusional parasitosis could arise from strategically placed lesions causing damage to the anatomical pathways, vascular compromise or to biochemical changes involving the neurotransmitter systems.

Diagnosis

Organic delusional disorders including delusional parasitosis share a common topography of lesions involving the subcortical limbic brain areas[86]. It is justified that an elderly person presenting with monosymptomatic delusional parasitosis is carefully evaluated for many can be expected to be suffering from cerebrovascular disease[81].

Treatment

Treatment begins with identifying the cause and treating it in patients presenting with delusional parasitosis associated with an organic disorder. Neuroleptics and antidepressants have been used and have helped to resolve the syndrome[86,87].

CLINICAL RELEVANCE—
NEUROPSYCHIATIC DISORDERS POST-STROKE

* Neuropsychiatric consequences of stroke include depression, mania, anxiety and psychiatric disorders.

* Primary depressive disorder has been divided into 'early onset' and 'late onset' (LOD) disorders. The late—onset is closely linked to clinical and neuroimaging evidence of cerebrovascular disease and there is a growing awareness of the influence of vascular based LOD and 'late onset mania'(LOM) lending support to distinct vascular subtypes.

* Neurotransmitter abnormalities occur and can be complex and more lately there has been considerable move towards embodying structural brain changes. in the causation of these disorders[30-32].

* Post-stroke depression is a serious disorder but is often overlooked and left untreated.

* Treatment principles are broadly similar to those currently used to treat non-organically ill patients.

* The term 'manic syndrome' in old age has its critics because of the high occurrence of medical and neurological conditions in old people with overall incidence of late—onset mania.

* The diagnosis of secondary mania is the presence of elevated or irritable mood together with at least two of the symptoms in the diagnosis of mania, symptoms duration of at least one week and no history of affective disorder and confusion.

* Lithium, valproic acid, carbamazepine, clonidine and neuroleptics may each be effective in the treatment of poststroke mania.

* Poststroke GAD can be diagnosed by using the DSM-IV symptom criteria[14].

* Cerebrovascular disease should be excluded in older persons with monosymptomatic delusional parasitosis.

* Neuropsychiatric and neurobehavioural disorders are important consequences of stroke and may impede recovery, rehabilitation and reduce quality of life.

References

1. Hickie I, Naismuth S, Ward PB et al. Reduced hippocampal volumes and memory loss in patients with early—and late—onset depression. *Br J Psychiatry* 2005; 186: 197-202.

2. Hickie I, Scott E, Wilhelm K, Brodaty H. Subcortical hyperintensities on magnetic resonance imaging in patients with severe depression-a longitudinal evaluation. *Biol Psychiatry* 1997; 42: 367-74.

3. Alexopolous GS, Meyers BS, Young RC et al. Clinically defined vascular depression. *Am J Psychiatry* 1997; 154: 497-501.

4. Mast BT, MacNeill SE, Litchenberg PA. Post-stroke and clinically defined vascular depression in geriatric rehabilitation. *Am J Geriatr Psychiatry* 2004; 12 (1): 84-92

5. Hickie IB. Reducing theburdens of depression: are we making progress in Australia? *Med J Aust* 2004; 181: S4-5.

6. Cummings JL. Organic delusions, phenomenology anatomical evaluation and review. *Br J Psychiatry* 1985; 146: 184-187.

7. Narushima K, Robinson RG. Stroke-related depression. *Curr Atheroscle Rep* 2002; 4(4): 296-303.

8. Schubert DS, Taylor C, Lee S et al. Physical consequences of depression in the stroke patient. *Gen Hosp Psychiatry* 1992; 14: 69-76.9

9. Whyte E M, Mulsant BH, Vandrbilt J et al. Depression after stroke: A prospective epidemiological study . . . *J Amer Geriatr Soc.* 2004; 52: 774-778.

10. Eastwood MR, Rifat SL, Nobbs H. Mood disorder following cerebrovascular accidents. *Br J Psychiatry* 1989; 154: 195-200.

11. DM, Finkelstein S. Delayed psychoses after right tempero-parietal stroke or trauma: relation to epilepsy. *Neurology* 1982; 32: 267-273.

12. Nagaratnam N, Pathma-Nathan N. Behavioural and psychiatric aspects of silent cerebral infarction. *Brit J Clin Pract.* 1997; 51: 160-163.

13. Bourgeous JA, Hilty DM, Chang CH, Servis ME. Post-stroke psychiatric syndromes: diagnosis and pharmacologic intervention *http://www.psychiatrictimes.com/display/article/10168/57491?verify+0 accessed 21/01/2010.*

14. Chemerinski E. Robinson RG. Neuropsychiatry of Stroke. *Psychsomatics* 2000; 41:5-14.

15. Schwartz JA, Peed NM, Brunberg JA et al. Depression in stroke rehabilitation. *Biol Psychiatry* 1993; 33(10): 694-9.

16. RM, Robinson RG Lipsey JR et al. The impact of poststroke depression on recovery in activities of daily living over a 2-year follow up. *Arch Neurol* 1990; 47:785-789.

17. Huffman JC, Stern TA. Poststroke neuropsychiatric symptoms and pseudoseizures: a discussion. *J Clin Psychiatry* 2003; 5(2): 85-88.

18. Carod-Artal F. Post-stroke depression (ii):its differential diagnsis, complications and treatment *Rev Neurol* 2006; 42(4): 238-44.

19. Robinson RG. Post-stroke de[ression, prevalence, diagnosis and treatment and disease

20. Robinson RG, PriceTR. Poststroke depression disorders: a follow-up study of 103 patients. *Stroke* 1982; 13: 635-41.

21. Starkstein SE, Robinson ER. Affective disorders in cerebrovascular disease. *Br J Psychiatry* 1989; 154: 170-182.

22. Robinson RG, Starkstein SE. Mood disorders folloing stroke: new findings and future directions *J Geriatr Psychiatry* 1989; 22(1): 1-15.

23. Hama S, Yamashita H, Shigenobu M et al. Poststroke affective or apathetic depression and lesion location:Left frontal lobe and bilateral basal ganglia. *Eur Arch Psychiatry Clin Neurosci.* 2007; 257: 149-152.

24. Santos M, Gold G, Kovari E et al. Differential impact of lacunes and microvascular lesions on poststroke depression. *Stroke* 2009; 40: 3557-3562.

25. House A, Dennis M, Warlow C et al. Mood disorders after stroke and their relation to lesion location *Brain* 1990; 113: 1113-29.

26. Sharpe M, Hawton K, House A. Mood disorders in long-term survivors of stroke associations with brain lesion location and volume. *Psychol Med* 1990;20:815-828.

27. Gottfries CG, Blennon K, Karisson I, Wallin A. The neurochemistry of vascular dementia. *Dementia* 1994; 5: 163-7.

28. Allard P, Englund E, Marcusson J. Reduced number of caudate nucleus dopamine uptake sites in vascular dementia. *Dementia Geriatr Cogn Disord* 1999; 10: 77-80.

29. Hickie IB, Naismuth SL, Norrie LM, Scott EM. Managing depression across the life cycle: new strategies for clinicians and their patients. *Int Med J* 2009; 39:720-723.

30. IB, Naismuth S, Ward PB. et al. Reduced hippocampal volumes and memory loss in patients with early—and late-onset depression. Br J Psychiatry 2005; 186: 197-202.

31. Naismuth SL, Hickie IB, Ward PB, et al. Impaired implicit sequence learning in depression: a probe for frontostriatal dysfunction? *Psychol Med* 2006; 36: 313-23.

32. Hickie B, Naismuth SL, Ward PB et al. Psychomotor slowing in older patients with major depression: relationships with blood flow in the caudate nucleus and white matter lesions. *Psychiatry Res* 2007;155: 211-20.

33. Krishnan KR, Hays JC, Blazer DG. MRI-defined vascular depression. *Am J Psychiatry* 1997; 154: 497-501.

34. Paranthaman R, Baldwin RC. Treatment of psychiatric syndromes due to cerebrvacular disease. *Int Rev Psychiatry* 2006; 18(5): 453-70.

35. Robinson RG, Schultz SK, Castillo C et al. Nortriptyline versus fluoxetine in the treatment of depression in short-term recovery after stroke: a placebo-controlled double blind study. *Am J Psychiatry* 2000; 157: 351-359.

36. Starkstein SE, Boston JD, Robinson RG. Mechanisms of mania after brain injury. 12 case reports and review of the literature. *J Nerv Ment.Dis.* 1988; 176:87-100.

37. T, Yamawaki S, Touhouda Y. Silent cerebral infarction in patients with late-onset mania. *Stroke* 1995; 26: 946-949.

38. Starkstein SE, Robinson ER. Affective disorders in cerebrovascular disease *Br J Psychiatry* 1989; 154: 170-182.

39. Herlihy Jr CE, Herlihy CE. Lithium and organic brain syndrome.*J Clin Psychiatry.* 1979; 40: 455 (Letter to Editor).

40. Jampala VC, Abrams R. Mania secondary to left and right hemispheric damage.*Am J Psychiatry.* 1983: 140: 1197-1199.

41. Turecki G, De Mari J, Porto JAD, Bipolar disorder following a laft ganglia stroke. *Br J Psychiatry.* 1993; 163:690.

42. Liu CY, Wang SJ, Fuh JL et al. Bipolar disorder following a stroke involving the left hemisphere. *Aust NZJ Psychiatry* 1996;30:688-691.

43. Fenn D, George K. Post-stroke mania in late life involving the left hemisphere *Aust NZJ Psychiatry* 1999;33:598-600.

44. Cummings JL. Organic delusions, phenomenology anatomical evaluation and reviews. *Br J Psychiatry* 1985; 146:184-197.

45. Starkstein SE, Fedoroff P, Berthier ML, Robinson RG. Manic depressive and pure manic states after brain lesions. *Biol Psychiatry* 1991; 29:149-158.

46. Bogousslavsky J, Ferrazziini M, Regli F et al. Manic delirium and frontal-like syndrome with paramedian infarction of the right thalamus. *J Neurol Neurosurg Psychiatry* 1988;51: 116-119.

47. Drake Jr ME, Pakalnis A, Phillips B. Secondary mania after ventral pontine infarction. J Neuropsychiatry *Clin Neurosci* 1990;2: 322-325.

48. Sandson TA, Daffner KR, Carvallio PA, Mesalum M. Frontal lobe dysfunction following infarction of the left-sided medial thalamus. *Arch Neurol* 1991; 48:1300-103,

49. Nagaratnam N, McNeill C, Gilhotra JS. Akinetic mutism and mixed transcortical aphasia following infarction of the left sided medial thalamus. *J Neurol Sci* 1999;163:70-73.

50. Clarke S, Assal G, Bogousslavsky J et al. Pure amnesia after unilateral left polar thalamic infarct. Topographic and sequential neurophysiological and metabolic (PET) correlations. *J Neurol Neurosurg Psychiatry* 1994;57:27-34.

51. Nagaratnam, Nagaratnam K. Frontal lobe dysfunction secondary mania and dementia syndrome following right posterior artery territory infarction. *Case Rep Clin Pract Rev.* 2005;6:

52. Nagaratnam N, Wong KK, Patel I. Secondary mania of vascular origin in elderly patients: A report of two clinical cases. *Arch Geront Geriatr.* 2006;43:223-232.

53. Alexander GE, De Long, Strick PL. Parallel organization of functionally segregated circuits linking basal ganglia and cortex. *J Neurosci* 1986;9: 357-381.

54. Cummings JL, Mendez MF. Secondary mania with focal cerebrovascular lesions. *Am J Psychiatry* 1884; 141:1084-1087.

55. Starkstein SE, Pearlson GB, Bosh J, Robinson RG. Mania after brain injury: controlled study of causative factors. *Arch Neurol* 1987;44: 1064-1073

56. Krauthammer C, Klerman GL. Manic syndromes associated with antecedent physical illness or drugs. *Arch Gen Psychiatry* 1978;35:1333-1339.

57. Levin M, Finkelstein S. Delayed psychosis after right tempero-parietal stroke or trauma: relation to epilepsy. *Neurology* 1982;32:267-273.

58. Evans DL, Byerly MJ, Greer RA. Secondary mmania: diagnosis and treatment *J Clin Psychiatry* 1995; 56:Suppl 3:31-7. (abstract).

59. Chemerinski E, Robinson RG et al Neuropsychiatry of stroke. *Psychosomatics* 2000;41:5-14.

60. Astrom M. Generalised anxiety disorder in stroke patients. *Stroke* 1996;27:270-275.

61. Burvill P, ohnson G, Jamrozik K et al. Risk factors for poststroke depression. *Int J Geriatr Psychiatry* 1997; 12: 219-225.

62. Castillo S, Starkstein SE, Fedoroff P et al. Generalised anxiety after stroke. *J Ner Ment Dis* 1993;181:100-106.

63. House A, Dennis M, Moridge L et al. Mood disorders in the year after first stroke. *Br J Psychiatry* 1991; 58:83-92.

64. Nagaratnam N. The development of panic attacks and social phobia *J Stroke Cerebrovasc Dis* 2000; 9(2):82-85.

65. LaplaneD, Levasseur M, Pillon Bet al. Obsessive-compulsive and other behavioural changes with bilateral basal ganglia lesions. A neuropsychological magnetic resonance imaging and positron tomography study. *Brain* 1989; 6: 237-255.

66. Robinson RG. The Clinical Neuropsychiatry of Stroke. New York. Cambridge University Press. 1998.

67. Rickels K, Schweizer EE. Current pharmacotherapy of anxiety and panic, in Psychophamacology: The Third Generation in Progress. Edited by Meltzer HY. New York, Raven 1987. pp 1193-1203.

68. Rabins PV, Sarkstein SE, Robinson Rg. Risk factors for developing atypical [schiziphreniform] psychosis following stroke. *J Neuropyschiatri Clin Neurosci* 1991; 2:6-9.

69. Levine DM, Finkelstein S. Delayed psychosis after right tempero-parietal stroke or trauma relation to epilepsy *Neurology* 1982; 32: 267-73.

70. Kumrai E, Ozturk O. Delusional state following acute stroke. *Neurology* 2004; 62:110-113.

71. Berthier M, Sarkstein SE. Acute atypical psychosis following right hemispheric stroke. *Acta Neurol Belg* 1987; 7: 125-31.

72. Bogousslavasky J, Ferrazzini M, Regli F et al Manic delirium and frontal like syndrome with paramedian infarction in the right thalamus. *J Neurol Neurosurg Psychiatry* 1988; 51: 116-119.

73. Soyka M, Naber G, Volcher A. Prevalence of delusional jealousy in different psychiatric disorders. An analysis of 93 cases.*Brit J Psychiatry* 1991; 159: 549-555.

74. Chin HF. Delusional jealousy in Chinese elderly psychiatric patients. *J Geriatr Psychiatry Neurol.* 1995; 8: 49-51.

75. Richardson ED, Malloy PF, Grace J. Othello syndrome secondary to right cerebrovascular infarction. *J Geriatr Psychiatry Neurol.* 1991; 4: 160-165.

76. Mitsuhata Y, Tsukagoshi H. Cerebellar infarctions presenting erotic delusions and delusion of jealousy. *Rinsho-Shingeigaku* 1992; 32: 1256-60.

77. Nagaratnam N, Gee R, Padma-Nathan N. Transient morbid jealousy following pontine infarction. *Eur J Int Med.* 1996; 7: 179-1

78. Leong GB, Silva AJ, Garza-Trevino et al. The dangers of persons with the Othello syndrome. *J Forensic Sci.*1994; 30: 1445-1454.

79. Trabet W. Delusional parasitosis: Studies on prevalence, classification and prognosis. *Hamburg/Saar.* 1993 (in German).

80. Heim M, Morgner J: Zur Problematik der chronischen taktilen Halluzinose. *Psychiatr Neurol Med Psychol* 1980; 32: 405-411.

81. Flynn FG, Cummings JL, Scheibel J. et al. Monosymptomatic delusions of parasitosis associated with ischaemic cerebrovascular disease. *J Geriatr Psychiat Neurol.*1989; 2: 134-138.

82. Peroutka SJ, Johmer BH, Kumer AJ et al. Hallucinations and delusions following a right temporoparietal occipital infarction. *John Hopkins Med J.*1982; 151: 181-185.

83. Cummings JL, Miller B, Hill MA et al. Neuropsychiatric aspects of multi—infarct dementia and dementia of the Alzheimer type. *Arch Neurol* 1987; 44: 389-393.

84. Nagaratnam N, O'Neile L. Deulsional parasitosis following occipito-temporal cerebral infarction. *Gen Hosp Psychiatry* 2000; 22: 129-132.

85. Cummings JL. Oganic psychosis. *Psychosomatics* 1988; 29: 16-26.

86. Andrews E, Bellard J, Walter-Ryan WG. Monosymptomatic hypochondriacal psychosis manifesting as delusions of infestation. Case studies of treatment with haloperidol. *J Clin Psychiatry* 1986; 47(4): 188.

87. Pylko T, Sicignan J. Nortriptline in the treatment of a monosymptomatic delusion. *Am J Psychiatry* 1985; 142: 1223.

15

Neurobehavioural

consequences of stroke

Introduction

Behaviour disorders are common in the elderly especially in those with dementia. More than half the patients admitted to nursing care facilities and a large majority of elderly admitted to acute care hospital have behaviour disorders. Changes in behaviour can affect the elderly in different ways. There are many reasons why a person's behavior can change.

This chapter describes the main neurobehavioural syndromes that accompany acute stroke. A wide variety of behavioural syndromes may occur after stroke depending on the location of the insult. They are distinct although there is overlap in their occurrence, neuropsychological and imaging findings. Numerous behavioural and emotional disorders such as aggressiveness, apathy, delirium, disinhibition, emotionalism following pathologic involvement of specific regions or functional systems have been described in post stroke patients. Behaviour disorders are important consequences of stroke and may impede recovery, rehabilitation and reduce quality of life.

Pathophysiology

The frontal lobes comprise one-third of our cerebral hemispheres but the literature has given little attention to unilateral strokes confined to the prefrontal cortex[1]. Asymptomatic cerebrovascular lesions are designated as silent cerebral infarction. Whether they are truly asymptomatic is unclear and the possibility of psychiatric subjective symptoms as manifestations in those with silent cerebral infarctions have been raised[2]. The clinical manifestations of frontal lobe pathology are protean; they depend not only on the size, side, depth and type but also on its interconnections.

Five segregated circuits had been proposed, each connecting the frontal lobe with the striatum, globus pallidus, substantia nigra, and thalamus[3]. Three of them are associated with three distinct frontal lobe neurobehavioural syndromes[4]. Irritability, tactlessness and unihibited behaviour are some features associated with the orbitofrontal syndrome. The dorsolateral involvement is characterized by reduced verbal and nonverbal fluency including perseveration[4]. Disinhibition has been observed with disorders of the subcortical structures, the caudate and thalamus[5].

De Long and Georgepolous[6] proposed a relationship between basal ganglia and the frontal cortical areas through a concept of 'motor' and 'complex' loops. Several functions mediated by both hemispheres interact with the limbic system. The limbic system has dense projections to the basal ganglia creating an integrated limbic-cortical system that mediates mood, motivation and motion[7]. A person's emotional behaviour is controlled by the limbic system in particular the amygdala, hypothalamus, septum and mesencephalon together with the reticular formation with frontal cortical interaction[7]. It is well known that the limbic system and the temporal are closely related to a number of psychological syndromes.

Frontal-subcortical circuits mediate many aspects of human behaviour[4]. A prototype of the circuit is—the frontal lobes have projections to the striatal structure with connections from the striatum to the globus pallidus and substantia nigra and from there to specific thalamic nuclei and finally back to the frontal lobes[4]. A wide range of behavioural alterations have been linked to dysfunction of the frontal-subcortical circuits and the character of the symptoms is probably associated with the site of the lesion although the nature of the association may be more complex.

Neurotransmitter systems include dopamine, acetylcholine and serotonin. Suitably placed lesions could cause an interruption by structural damage or by interference with transmitter systems. Overactivity of the dopaminergic pathways may play an important role in the causation of mania and serotonin can play a role in the regulation of mood. Instability in behaviors such as sexual disinhibition and aggression can result from decreased release of GABA.

I. ACUTE CONFUSIONAL STATE (ACUTE DELIRIUM)

Introduction

Acute confusional state (ACS) is a disorder that reflects disturbance of global attention and attention directed disorders[8]. Elderly people are particularly vulnerable to acute confusion. Altered behavior in the elderly may be the first indication of acute confusional state (ACS) and violent behavior can also be a part of the acute confusional state or delirium in the acute phase of the ictus. Manifestation of acute confusional state is a wide spectrum from one of apathy, lethargy to one of agitation. Most patients with acute confusion suffer from a reversible toxic, infectious or metabolic disorder. It is well known that focal lesions in the brain can give rise to acute confusional state.

Incidence prevalence epidemiology

ACS occurs in one fourth of stroke patients over the age of 40 years[9]. Stroke is known to be a predisposing factor for delirium and there are conflicting results with prevalence estimates ranging from 13-48% [10] depending on the population studied and the definition of ACS [9]. In a study of 83 patients after ischaemic supratentorial stroke ACS was seen in 35 (42%)[11]. More than half (25/41) the patients with infarct in the right middle cerebral artery territory presented with ACS [12]. Delirium can be a presenting feature in a few patients and can complicate the clinical course of acute stroke in upto 48% of cases [13].

Pathophysiology

It is well known that lesions in the non-dominant hemisphere, in the territories of the middle cerebral[14;15] and posterior cerebral arteries[16] can cause ACS. Those involving the cortex have been well described but those subcortical are less clear and the lesions existed in different sites for each patient reported, the corona radiata above the head of the caudate, the anterior limb of the internal capsule, caudate nucleus, centrum semi-ovale and deep parietal[17]. Anteromedial thalamic stroke[18], infarction in the interpeduncular profundus territory[19] and in the genu of the internal capsule [20] and in the anterior border zones[21] have given rise to confusional syndrome.

There are several observations upholding the hypothesis that multiple neurotransmitter abnormalities occur in ACS [22]. More important ones being acetylcholine (ACh) and dopamine. In support of the role of ACh in the pathogenesis of ACS, anti-cholinergic medications (atropine) or drugs with anticholinergic activity (anti-psychotics, anti-depressives, bladder relaxants among others) are known to cause ACS and those with impaired cholinergic transmission as in Alzheimer's disease are particularly susceptible to ACS. There is also an increase in dopaminergic activity in ACS and a reciprocal relationship exists between cholinergic and dopaminergic activity [22]. Patients with Parkinson's disease treated with L-dopa and or dopamine agonists are frequently seen to become delirious.

Delirium has been associated with disruption of the cortisol and beta-endorphin circadian rhythm. Stroke patients had a higher cortisol levels after dexamethasone than the elderly healthy control population[11]. According to Gustafson et al[11] it is possible and should be considered that hypercortisolism is involved in the pathophysiology of confusion caused by acute stroke. A study of right hemispheric stroke patients by Olsson et al[23] found possible disturbance at different sites of the hypothalamic-pituitary—adrenal axis, with increased levels of dexamethasone—cortisol levels which could be significantly correlated to the presence of ACS with extensive limb paresis.

Diagnosis

Most stroke patients develop delirium at stroke onset and this may remain for appreciable period. Predictors for ACS in stroke patients include severity of the stroke, previous ACS, older age, left-sided lesions and treatment with anti-cholinergics[24], haemorrhagic stroke and ischaemic stroke in the anterior circulation[25]. It is related to unsafe swallowing on admission, poor vision pre-stroke, and reduced C-Reactive Protein on admission[26].

Treatment

Early recognition and treatment is vital. The treatment is aimed at correcting the underlying abnormality causing the confusion. Currently there is no reliable way of predicting who is at risk of developing ACS. Apart from the known precipitating factors the onset of delirium poststroke is likely to depend on a number of factors, such as the location of the lesion, severity of the stroke, type of stroke and the degree of cerebral hypoperfusion and oedema together with any medical complications such as infection, aspiration pneumonia[10].

The next step is directed towards controlling the agitation and disruptive behaviours. They may require the use of psychotropic drugs such as respiridone and tradazone. Non-pharmacological interventions are the key measures in the management of ACS. Behavioural approaches to management are preferable if effective. Concurrently supportive and restorative care should be provided. Fluid and nutritional needs attended to. Patient should be monitored day and night and there should be continuity of care by the staff. ACS is a marker of poor prognosis. It carries a high mortality and morbidity and longer stay in hospital.

II. MUTISM, APATHY, ABULIA

Introduction

Akinetic mutism (AM), abulia and apathy are terms that have been used to describe behavioral abnormalities relating to reduced activity and slowness. Apathy is characterized as lack of feeling and emotional unconcern. AM is characterized by marked reduction including facial expression, gestures and speech output but with some degree of alertness.

Incidence prevalence epidemiology

Apathy is common and a frequent finding in patients with acute stroke lesions. In the Sydney Stroke Study in the 3-month follow up depression was only present in 10% of the stroke patients, apathy only in 23% and both apathy and depression in 7%[27].

Pathophysiology

AM has been reported following lesions in the the frontal lobe (cingulated gyrus, supplementary motor area and the anterior dorsal lateral border zone), basal ganglia (caudate and putamen) mesencephalon and thalamus[28,29]. AM has been reported after involvement of either cerebral hemispheres[29,30]. Unilateral lesions are said to give rise to transient AM and bilateral lesions to more prolonged AM. Prolonged abulia has followed putaminal haemorrhage[31]. There is a wide network of anatomical structures involved which included the frontal lobe and subcortical structures. Integration of these structures is by way of the frontosubcortical circuits and AM could result from damage to the frontal lobe and or interruption of the frontosubcortical circuitry. There is slightly a higher rate of apathy with right hemispheric strokes (31.8%) than strokes involving the left hemisphere in one study[32]. The common pathophysiology of AM appears to be involving the mesocortical dopaminergic system with successful reports of treatment with dopamine agonists[33]. Acetylcholine, dopamine and to a lesser extent serotonin appear to be the most important neurotransmitters involved in apathy[34].

Diagnosis

The clinical features of AM correspond more closely to the functional anatomy of the brain regions involved than to the pathology. The important risk factors for apathy reported are older age, poor cognitive status, low functional status in stroke patients[35]. Apathy is often associated with functional impairment and cognitive deficits. It is often confused with depression. Neuroimaging correlates of depression and apathy are different. It is important to recognize the distinction as there treatment differs [36].

Treatment

Apathy responds well to psychostimulants. In AM if the causative lesion is in the frontal lobe successful treatment with L-dopa or dopamine agonists such as bromocriptine had been reported[33]. Three cases with AM had been successfully treated with intramuscular olanzapine and the authors believe this is due to olanzapine's indirect elevation of dopamine in the mesocortical pathway[37].

III. AGGRESSION OR INABILITY TO CONTROL ANGER

Introduction

The behaviours reported consisted of a constellation of symptoms, physical, verbal or sexual aggression, or anxiety or both, agitation, pacing, wandering or hyperactive vocalization. Several investigators have pointed out that such verbal outbursts, agitation, screaming and wandering are a continuum of severity of hyperactive behaviour.

Incidence prevalence epidemiology

In a study of 145 patients after stroke 47 (32%) had inability to control anger and aggression[38].

Pathophysiology

Aggressive conduct has been associated with specific localization of ischaemic lesions—in the cingulum, frontal and temporal lobes and the hypothalamus. It involves the fronto-lenticular-capsular pontine base areas[38]. The frontal lobe and frontal subcortical circuitry play an important role in the occurrence of aggression and agitation Hyperactivity, disinhibition, impulsiveness and disability are behaviours associated with orbitofrontal lesions and can be explained by frontocortical abnormality[21]. Aggressive behaviours have also been related to the presence of brain lesions in the paralimbic areas of the temporal lobe[39]and prefrontal cortex[40]. Aggressive behaviour is a rare ccurrence with acute posterior cerebral artery territory stroke. Severity of the stroke, psychopathology and neurobiologic factors appear to contribute to irritable and aggressive behaviour in stroke patients[41].

Various neurotransmitters have been associated with aggressive behaviour, an increase in acetylcholine and cathecolamines and a decrease in GABA and 5-hydroxyindolacetic acid. Abnormalities of the serotonergic system may be associated with impulsive and violent behaviour. There are reports of a specific subtype of major depressive disorder characterized by anger and aggressive behaviour associated with a dysfunction of the serotonergic system[42,43]. It is possible that interruption of the serotonergic pathway by frontal lobe damage could contribute to the pathophysiology of both depression and violent behaviour[44].

Diagnosis

Inability to control anger (ICAA) was closely related to motor dysfunction, emotional incontinence and dysarthria and ICAA appears to be one of the major behavioural symptoms in patients with stroke[38]. ICCA can seriously interfere with rehabilitation and cause considerable stress to family, health care providers and other patients[45].

Treatment

It has been shown that fluoxetine reduced poststroke anger levels[46]. Reductions in depression and reductions in aggression and irritability in patients with stroke have followed pharmacological interventions[47].

IV. HYPERSEXUALITY AND INAPPROPRIATE SEXUAL BEHAVIOR

Introduction

The continuance of sexual expression in the elderly as age advances is well recognized. The sexually related behaviors include cuddling, touching of the genitals, sexual remarks, propositioning, grabbing and groping, use of obscene language and masturbating without shame[48,49]. Sexual inappropriate behaviors remain highly controversial and labeling them as 'diseased' or an illness may have enormous individual, cultural and medico-legal implications.

Incidence, prevalence and epidemiology

Hypersexuality following stroke has been less frequently reported compared to hyposexuality after stroke which is a common problem. Little less than half of the 41 patients with sexually inappropriate behaviour were in nursing homes and the remaining in the community and more commonly in the subjects of vascular etiology, 53.7% had vascular dementia[50].

Pathophysiology

Computed tomography has revealed infarction in the frontal lobe, temporoparietal, thalamus, caudate and lentiform nucleus[49]. There are reports of hypersexuality following strokes in the region of the basal ganglia[51]. Although in many the lesions were non-frontal in some the symptomatology were suggestive of frontal involvement. Many exhibited in addition aggression, agitation and irritability. Mongo et al[52] described three patients who demonstrated hypersexuality and deviant sexual behaviour after stroke. All three had temporal lobe lesions on CT scan and all had a history of poststroke seizure activity.

Kluver and Bucy[53] described behavioural changes following bilateral temporal lobectomies in rhesus monkeys.

Diagnosis

The changes include increased sexual activity, antisocial behaviour and changes in dietary habits[53]. Damage to the limbic system and its connections in all probability plays an important role.

Treatment

Patients who exhibit hypersexual behaviour following stroke may benefit with behavioural interventions. In some, simple explanation and such techniques as distraction, redirection and removal of 'sexual triggers' may be sufficient[54]. There is some evidence that antidepressants, anticonvulsants and antipsychotics maybe useful.

V. EMOTIONALISM, PATHOLOGICAL CRYING AND CATASTROPHIC REACTION

Introduction

A common denominator to all three is crying. In emotionalism the crying is congruent with mood and it is uncontrollable[55]. Pathological crying is uncontrollable episodes of crying and which is not a primary disturbance of feeling but a disorder of expression[56]. In catastrophic reaction the crying is brought on when a task is not possible and giving up due to neurological deficit (left hemispheric lesions) or by indifference (right hemispheric lesions)[55]. In catastrophic reaction there are outbursts of anger, aggressiveness, anxiety and frustration[55]. Pathological crying is also referred to as emotional lability, pseudobulbar effect and more recently involuntary emotional expression disorder (IEED)[57]. Although they share some symptoms in common they are distinct entities[58].

Incidence prevalence and epidemiology

10-15% of post-stroke patients manifest pseudobulbar effect[59]. Emotionalism was reported in 13 0f 89 patients (15%) at one month, 25 of 119 (21%) at 6 months and 12 of 112 (11%) at 12 months after stroke[60].

Pathophysiology

An understanding of the underlying mechanisms will assist in potential and effective treatments. Pathological crying has resulted from bilateral hemispheric, bilateral pontine[61] and from left anterior choroidal artery infarction[62,63]. Pseudo-bulbar patients with crying or laughter have bilateral lesions. There is a strong association between lateralization and emotional processes, in those with the larger lesion on the left there is crying and in those with right there is laughter[64]. Catastrophic reaction occurs with left hemispheric lesions and aphasia [55].

A series of parallel circuits link the frontal lobe with the subcortical structures[65] and neurotransmitters like serotonin, acetyl choline and dopamine have a modulating role. It had been postulated that serotonergic neurotransmission plays an important role in poststroke pathological crying[66]. A single lesion suitably placed in the sertononergic pathway could give rise to pathological crying.

Diagnosis

Poststroke pathological crying can be distressing to the patient[66,67] resulting in family and caregiver stress. The differential diagnosis includes pseudobulbar palsy, frontal lobe lesions due to traumatic injury among others. The crying or laughter cannot be stopped voluntarily in patients with pseudo-bulbar palsy and the patients have a feeling of normal emotions. In pseudo-bulbar palsy, the cortico-bulbar motor pathways are interrupted resulting in release from cortical control of the reflex mechanisms for facial expression[68]. There is weakness of voluntary facial muscles with increased jaw jerk and results from bilateral lesions[64] but could result from unilateral lesions on either side. Unlike in pseudobulbar palsy frontal lobe disorders with true emotional labilities do not have appropriate internal emotional feeling.

Treatment

It is reasonable to assume that selective serotonin reuptake inhibitors would be useful to control the symptoms in patients with pathological crying. Amitriptyline, nortryptyline, l-dopa[67], citalopram[66], fluoxetine[67,48] and paroxetene[62] have given rise to considerable amelioration of symptoms. There has been reports that emotionalism may respond to tricyclic antidepressants and levadopa[69-72]. Catastrophic reaction occurs frequently in patients with nonfluent aphasia after stroke. It is adviced that during rehabilitation language testing and therapy should not be pushed too hard in an already frustrated and depressed patient[73]. In a single patient with post stroke pathological laughing and crying, lamotrigine a antiepileptic drug with antidepressant and mood-stabilizing properties had a beneficial effect. Lamotrigine was given at the dose of 50 mg initially and gradually increased to 100mg a day over 4-weeks and had significant and rapid recovery in both components, laughing and crying[74].

VI. DISINHIBITION SYNDROMES

Introduction

Starkstein and Robinson [75] described 5 aspects of disinhibition syndrome namely motor (eg hyperactivity), instinctive (eg hypersexuality and hyperphagia), emotional (eg euphoria and elation), intellectual (eg flight of ideas) and sensory (eg hallucinations).

Incidence prevalence and epidemiolgy

There has been no precise reports on epidemiological studies on disinhibition[76].

Pathophysiology

Lesions in specific brain areas could give rise to disinhibition syndromes ranging from inappropriate social behaviour to full blown mania. There is a significant association between disinhibition syndromes and dysfunction of the orbito-frontal and baso-temporal cortices of the right hemisphere[75]. Disinhibition has been observed with disorders of the subcortical structures, the caudate and the thalamus[5]. Abyeck et al[76]reported that disinhibition was significantly associated with supratentorial lesions and in contrast to other authors they found no differences between left and right hemisphere localization.

Nearly all lesions producing disinhibition and secondary mania have involved the right hemisphere[77]. In the 11 all male poststroke patients with sexually—related behaviours the CT scan showed lesions located in the left putamen, right parieto-temporal, right parietal, right thalamus, left orbito-frontal, left dorso-lateral, left mescencephalo-thalmic, bilateral lesions in one, with right posterior cerebral artery infarction in one and left middle cerebral artery infarction[48,49].

Diagnosis

Shulman[78] drew attention to the close resemblance of mania to the disinhibition syndromes. In two studies of five and six patients respectively, with sexually disinhibited behaviours following stroke all had two or more of the core features of mania, namely elated mood, aggression, irritability and hostility, decreased sleep, impulsive behaviour, overtalkativeness, restlessness and increased activity and activity with poor attention[49,78]. Two patients described by Mongo et al [52] exhibited mood changes, deviant sexual behaviour and hyperphagia. In a study of 12 patients with behaviour related problems because of the stereotyped patterns in the location of the lesions they were grouped accordingly. The groups were predominantly orbitofrontal, deep white matter and border zones. Hyperactvity, disinhibition, irritability and impulsiveness with orbitofrontal lesions, the second group manifested predominantly cognitive impairment and the third group, the predominant symptom was a confusional state. In this study the symptoms overlapped. Each patient had different distribution of the deficits [49]. Likewise many of the changes associated with prefrontal lesions often overlap with the range of human behaviour[1]. According to Strub et al,[79] there is no unitary behavioural correlation of symptoms with frontal lobe damage. Involvement of the lateral portions of the frontal lobe usually gives rise to the apathetic components of the frontal lobe syndromes, but a bilateral anterior communicating artery aneurysm rupture provided the same symptoms with mesial and orbital involvement[80].

Treatment

Spiegel et al [79] described three cases of disinhibition and aggression involving the frontal subcortical circuits treated successfully with carbamazepine. In one the lesion was in the internal capsule. In the second there was a fronto-parietal haematoma and the third had an extensive subarachnoid haemorrhage involving the cortices and right frontal subcortical white matter.

CLINICAL RELEVANCE—Neurobehavioural syndromes

* A wide variety of behavioural disorders may occur after stroke depending on the location of the insult.
* Neurobehavioural disorders such as aggressiveness, apathy, mutism confusional state, emotionalism and disinhbition have been described post-stroke.
* Delirium can be a presenting feature in a few patients and can complicate the clinical course of acute stroke in upto 48% of cases.
* Early recognition and treatment is vital.
* Important to look for underlying causes (brain imaging tp look for focal lesions) and most of the time management is supportive.
* Apathy is common and a frequent finding in patients with acute stroke lesions.
* Inability to control anger (ICAA) was closely related to motor dysfunction, emotional incontinence and dysarthria and ICAA appears to be one of the major behavioural symptoms in patients with stroke[38].
* Patients who exhibit hypersexual behaviour following stroke may benefit with behavioural interventions.
* Poststroke pathological crying can be distressing to the patient resulting in family and caregiver stress.
* There is close resemblance of mania to the disinhibition syndromes.
* Behavioural disorders are important consequences of stroke as they may impede recovery, rehabilitation and reduce quality of life.

References

1. Mesulam MM. Frontal cortex and behaviour. *Ann Neurol*.1986; 19(4): 320-25.
2. Fujikawa T, Yamawaki S, Touhouda Y. Silent cerebral infarctions in patients with late-onset mania. *Stroke* 1995; 26(6): 946-949.
3. Alexander GE, Delaney MR, Sbruck PL. Parallel organizations of functionally segregated circuits linking basal ganglia and cortex. *Ann Rev. Neuroscience* 1990; 9: 357-381.
4. Cummings JL. Frontal-subcortical circuits and human behaviour. *Arch Neurol* 1993; 50 (8): 873-880.
5. Gentilini M, De Renzi E, Crisi G. Bilteral paramedian thalamic artery infarcts: report of eight cases. *J Neurol Neurosurg Psychiatry* 1987; 50: 900-909.
6. De Long HR, Georgepolous AP. Motor functions of the basal ganglia as revealed by studies of single cell activity in the behaving primate. *Arch Neurol* 1979; 24: 131-140.
7. Nauta WJH. Limbic innervation of striatum. In: Friedhoff AJ, Chase TN (Eds), Giles de la Tourette syndrome. Raven Press, New York. pp 41-48.
8. Mesulam MM. Attention confusional state and neglect. In Mesulam MM. Principles of behavioural neurology. Philadelphia. 1985.
9. Henon H, Lebert F, Duricu I et al. Confusional state in stroke relating to pre-existing dementia patient characteristics and outcome. *Stroke* 1999; 30: 773-779.
10. McManus J, Pathansali R, Stewart R et al,. Delrium poststroke. *Age Ageing* 2007; 36(60:613-618.
11. Gustafson Y, Olsson T, Asplund K, Hagg E. Acute confusional state (delirium) soon after stroke is associated with hypercorticolism. *Cerebrovasc Dis*. 1993; 3:33-38.
12. Mori E, Yamadori A. Acute confusional state and acute agitated delirium. *Arch Neurol* 1987; 44(11): 1139-1143.
13. Ferro JM, Caeiro L Verdelho A. Delrium in acute stroke. *Current opinion in Neurology*. 2002; 15(1): 51-55.
14. Mesulam MM, Lekoff SE, Wetie et al. Acute confusional; state with right sided cerebral artery infarctions. *J Neurol Neurosurg Psychiatry*. 1976; 39: 84-95.
15. Caplan LR, Kelly M. Kase CS et al. Infarction of the right middle cerebral artery. *Neurology* 1986; 56: 1015-28.
16. Devinsky O, Bear D, Volpe BT. Confusional states following posterior cerebral artery infarction. *Arch Neurol* 1988; 45: 601-606.
17. Nagaratnam N, Nagaratnam K. Subcortical origins of acute confusional states. *Eur J Int Med* 1995; 6: 55-58.
18. Santamaria J, Blesa R, Tolosa ES. Confusional syndrome in thalamic stroke. *Neurology* 1984; 34: 1618.
19. Graff-Radford NR, Eslinger PJ, Damasio AR, Yamada T. Non-haemorrhagic infarction of the thalamus: behavioural, anatomic and physiologic correlates. *Neurology* 1984; 34: 14-23.

20. Tatemichi TK, Desmond DW, Prohovnik I et al. Confusion and memory loss from capsular genu infarction: a thalamocortical disconnection syndrome? *Neurology* 1992; 42: 1966-79.

21. Nagaratnam N, Bou-Haider P, Leung H. Confused and disturbed behaviour in the elderly following silent frontal lobe infarction. *Am J Alz Dis Other Dementias*. 2003; 18(6): 331-335.

22. Alagaikrishnan K, BlanchetteP. Delirium. *Delirium eMedicine Psychiatry. http://www.emedicine.mediscape.com/article/28890-overview* accessed 16/02/2010.

23. Olsson T, Marklund N, Gustafson Y et al. Abnormalities at different levels of the hypothalamic-pituitary-adrenocortical axis early after stroke. *Stroke* 1992; 23(11): 1573-1576.

24. Gustafson Y, Olsson T, Erikson S et al. Acute confusional state (delirium) in stroke. *Cerebrovasc Dis* 1991; 1 257-264.

25. Dostovic Z, Smajlovic D, Sinanovic D, Vidovic M. et al. Duration of delirium in the acute stage of stroke. *Acta Clin Croat* 2008; 48: 13-17.

26. McManus J, Pathasali R, Hassan H et al. *Age Ageing*. Advance Aces published Aptril 2009.

27. Barclay L. Apathy is independent of depression after stroke. website: *http://www.medscape.com/viewarticle/469698.* accessed on 16/02/2010.

28. Nagaratnam N, McNeil C, Gilhotra JS. Akinetic mutism and mixed transcortica; aphasia following left thalamo-mesencephalic infarction. *J Neurol Sci* 1999; 163:70-73.

29. Nagaratnam N, Nagaratnam K, Ng K, Diu P. Akinetic mutism following stroke *J Clin Neurosci* 2004;11(1):25-30.

30. Bougouslavksy J, Regli F, Assal G. Acute transcortical mixed aphasia. A carotid occlusion syndrome with pial and watershed infarcts. *Brain* 1988; 11: 631-641.

31. Nagaratnam N, Fanello S, Gopinath S, Goodwin A. Prolonged abulia following putaminal haemorrhage. *J Stroke Cerebrovasc* Dis 2001; 10: 273-290.

32. Marin RS, Firinciogullari S, Biedrzckr DC. Group differences in the relationship between apathy and depression. *J Nerv Ment Dis* 1994; 182: 235-237.

33. Trzepacz P, Meagler D. Delirium in Textbook of Psychosomatic Medicine; 1st Ed. Edited by Levenson JL, Arlington VA. Americal Psychiatric Publishers Inc 2005pp 91-130.

34. van Reekum R, Stuss DT, Ostrander L. Apathy: Why care? *J Neuropsychiatry Clin Neurosci* 2005; 17: 7-19.

35. NE, Fellows LK, Scott SE. A longitudinal view of apathy and its impct on stroke. *Stroke* 2009; 40: 3299-3307.

36. Brodaty H, Sachdev P, Withall A et al. Frequency and clinical neuropsychiatric and neuroanatomic correlations of apathy after stroke. The Sydney Stroke Study. *Psychol Med* 2005; 35: 1707-1710.

37. Spiegel DR, Casello DP, Collender DM, Dhadwal N. Treatment with akinetic mutism with intramuscular olanzapine: A case series. *J Neuropsychiatry Clin Neurosci* 2008; 20: 93-95.

38. Kim JS, Choi S, Kum SV, Seo YC. Inability to control anger or aggression after stroke. *Neurology* 2002; 58 (7): 1106-8

39. Tonkongy JM. Violence and temporal lobe lesions; head CT and MRI. *J Neuropsychiatr Clin Neurosci* 1991; 3: 189-196 (abstract).

40. Grafman J, Schwab K, Warden D et al. Frontal lobe injuries, violence and aggression. A report of the Vietnam head injury study. *Neurology*. 1996; 46: 231-30.

41. Chan KI, Canpayo A, Mosu DJ et al. Aggressive behaviour ib patients with stroke: association with psychopathy and results of antidepressant treatment on aggression. *Arch Phys Med Rehabil* 2006; 87 (6): 793-8.

42. Yudotsky SC, Silver JM, Jackson W et al. The overt aggresive scale for the objective rating of verbal and physical aggression. *Am J Psychiatr* 1988; 143: 38-39.

43. Mysiw WJ, Sandek ME. The agitated brain injured patient. Pathophysiology and treatment. *Arch Phys Med Rehabil* 1997;78: 213-220.

44. Faun JR, Uomoto JM, Katon WJ. Serataline in treatment of major depression following mild traumatic brain injury. *J Neuropsychol Clin Neurosci* 2000, 12: 226-232

45. Santos CS, Ciero L, Ferros JM et al. Anger hostility and aggression in the first days of acute stroke. *Eur J Neurol* 2006; 13(4): 351-8.

46. Choi-Kwon S, Han SW, Kwon SU et al. Fluoxetine treatment in poststroke depression: emotional incontinence and anger proness: A double blind placebo-controlled study. *Stroke* 2006;17:156-161.

47. Chan KL, Campayo A, Moser DJ et al. Aggressive behavior in patients with stroke: Association with psychoplathology and results antidepressant treatment on aggression. *Arch Phys Med Rehabil* 2006;87:773-778.

48. Nagaratnam N, Tse A, Lim R et al. Aberrant sexual behavior following stroke. *Eur J Int Med* 1998; 9: 207-209.

49. Nagaratnam N, Gayagay Jr. Hypersexuality in nursing care facilities-a descriptive study. *Arch Geront Geriatr* 2002; 35: 195-203.

50. Alagiakrishnan K, Lim D, Brahim A. Sexual inappropriate behaviour in demented elderly people. *Postgrad Med* J 2005; 81: 453-465.

51. Libman RB, Wirkowski EJ. Hypersexuality and stroke: A role for the basal ganglia? *Cerebrovasc Dis* 1996; 6: 111-113(abstract).

52. Monga TN, Monga M, Raina MS, Hardjasudarma M. Hypersexuality in stroke. *Arch Phys Med Rehabil* 1986; 67(6): 415-7 [Abstract].

53. Kluver H, Bucy PC. Preliminary analysis of temporal lobes in monkeys. *Arch Neurol Psychiatry* 1939; 42: 979-1000.

54. Kellogg-Spadt, Browes C. Hypersexual behavior following stroke. *http:// www.Sexualityandaging.com/wp-content/uploads/2010/02/Bowes_Kellogg-St. retrieved* on 20/09/2012.

55. Carota A, Berneya A, Aybeck S. A prospective study of predictors of poststrole depression. *Neurology* 2005;64:428-438.

56. Parvizi J, Anderson SW, Martin CO. Pathological laughing and crying. A link to the cerebellum. *Brain* 2001;124(():1708-1713. Doi: 10.1093/brain/124.9.1708

57. Cummings JL, Arciniegas DB, Brooks BR. et al. Defining and diagnosing involuntary emotional expression disorder. *CNS Spectr.* 2006; 11(6): 1-7.

58. Levenson JL. Psychiatric Issues in Neurology, Part1: Stroke. *Primary Psychiatry* 2007;14(7):39-40.

59. Huffman JC, Stern TA. Poststroke neuropsychiatric symptoms and pseudoseizures: A discussion. *J Clin Psychiatry* 2003; 5(2):85-88.

60. House A, Dennis M, Molyneux A et al. Emotionalism after stroke. *Brit Med* J 1989; 298(6679):941-994.

61. Anderson G, Ingeman-Nielson M, Vestergaard K et al. Pathoanatomic correlation between pathologic crying and damage to brain areas involved in serotonergic neurotransmission. *Stroke* 1994; 25: 1050-1052.

62. Derex L Ostrowsky K, Nighoghossian N et al. Severe pathological crying after left anterior choroidal artery infarct—reversibility with paroxetine treatment. *Stroke* 1997; 28: 1464-1466.

63. Nagaratnam N, Wong V, Jeyaratnam D. Left anterior choroidal artery infarction and uncontrollable crying. *J Stroke Cerebrovasc Dis* 1998;7: 263-264.

64. Sackeim HA, Greenberg MS, Weiman AL et al. Hemispheric asymmetry in the expression of positive and negative conditions. *Arch Neurol* 1982; 39: 210-218.

65. Alexander GE, De Long MR, Strick PL. Parralel organization of functionally segregated circuits linking basal ganglia and cortex. *Ann Rev Neurosci* 1986; 9: 357-381.

66. Anderson G, Vestergaard K, Riis JO. Poststroke pathological crying treated with the selective reuptake inhibitor citalopram. *Lancet* 1993; 342: 837-839.

67. Hanger HC. Emotionalism after stroke. *Lancet* 1993; 342: 1235-123663.

68. Rinn WE. The neuropsychology of facial expression: A review of neurological and psychological mechanisms of producing facial expressions. *Psychol Bull* 1984; 95:52-77.

69. Schiffer RB, Cash J, Herndon RM. Treatment of emotional lability with low dosage tricyclic antidepressants. *Psychosomatics.* 1983; 24: 1094-6.

70. Schiffer RB, Herndon RM, Radick R. Treatment of pathological laughing and weeping with amitryptline. *N Engl J Med* 1985; 312: 1480-2.

71. Wolf JK, Santana HB, Thorpy M. Treatment of 'emotional incontinence' with levodopa. *Neurology* 1979: 29: 1455-6.

72. Udaka F, Yamao S, Nagatta H et al. Pathologic laughing and grinning treated with levodopa. *Arch Neurol* 1979;29:1455-6.

73. Chemerinski E, Robinson RG. Neuropsychiatry of Stroke. *Psychosomatics* 2000; 41: 5-14.

74. Ramasubbu R. Lamotrigine: Treatment for poststroke pathological laughing and crying. *Clin Neuropharmcol* 2003; 25(5): 233-5.

75. Starkstein SE, Robinson ER. Mechanism of disinhibition after brain lesions. *J Nerv Ment Dis* 1997;185:108-114.

76. Aybek S, Carota A, Ghika-Schmid F et al. Emotions in acute stroke: The Lausanne Emotion in Stroke Study *Cognitive and Behavioral Neurol* 2005;18(1): 37-44.

77. Steffens DC, Krishnan KRR. Structural imaging and mood disorders. Recent findings, implications for classification and future directions. *Biol Psychiatry* 1998; 43: 705-712.

78. Shulman KI. Mania in old age: A neuropsychiatric syndrome. *Geriatrics Aging* 2004;7: 34-37.

79. Strub RI. Frontal lobe syndrome in a patient with bilateral globus pallidus lesions. *Arch Neurol* 1989; 46(9): 1024-1027.

80. Wilson SAK. Disorders of mobility and of muscle tone with special reference to corpus striatum. *Lancet* 1985; 9: 357-381.

81. Spiegel DR, Burgess J, Samuels D et al. Disinhibition due to disruption of the orbitofrontal circuit treated successfully with carbamazepine: a case series. *J Neuropsychiatr & Clin Neurosci* 2009;21(3): 323-327.

16

STROKE AND VASCULAR COGNITIVE IMPAIRMENT/VASCULAR DEMENTIA

Introduction

The misconception that cerebral atherosclerosis with resultant chronic hypoperfusion is the cause of organic dementia prevailed in the 1950s. Vascular disease giving rise to relatively large infarcts enough to damage a sufficient volume of the brain causing dementia was termed multi-infarct dementia[1]. The term vascular dementia (VaD) is not only the traditional multi-infarct dementia but has a broader connotation and embraces all others due to different vascular mechanisms and changes in the brain with different causes and manifestations[2]. However, according to Lodder[3] the terms 'vascular dementia' or 'poststroke dementia' 'are not diagnoses but concepts that have resulted from the procedure of medical consensus'. It has been suggested that VaD should be re-defined with greater consideration to the identification of distinct vascular mechanisms in the development of dementia[4]. Nevertheless irrespective of the definition, VaD remains within the spectrum of cerebrovascular disease. In view of the complexity of the mechanisms likely to be responsible for VaD several factors such as sociodemographic factors, neuroimaging features and comorbidities should be taken into account[5].

Currently the term vascular cognitive impairment (VCI) has been proposed. It includes a wide spectrum of cognitive declines ranging from mild deficits in one or more cognitive domains to a broad dementia—like syndrome[6]. It is a preferred term for it encompasses the complex interactions between vascular risk factors, cerebrovascular disease etiology and cellular changes within the brain and cognition[6]. In this chapter the terms VaD and VCI are interchangeable.

Incidence prevalence and epidemiology

The very elderly are at the highest risk for cognitive impairment and dementia and stroke is among the risk factors[7]. Dementia (VaD) is probably the second commonest cause of dementia after Alzheimer's disease (AD) in the Western countries but may be more common than AD after the age of 85 years[8] and in countries like Japan, China and Russia[9]. Some believe that Lewy body dementia (LBD) may be more common than VaD[10,11]. Little more than quarter of the patients with acute stroke develop dementia[12,13]. Stroke and dementia increase exponentially with age and hence there may be a significant overlap between VaD and AD and at very high levels may level off. It is much more common in men before the age of 75 years and the prevalence is higher in women after the age of 80 years[14,15]. Men are said to be at a higher risk of VaD than women and is a reverse of AD[16]. Studies have shown that 30% of the stroke survivors over the 75 years suffer from dementia[5].

Pathophysiology

Traditionally VaD had been characterized as having a "patchy" pattern of cognitive deficits but this patchy pattern is associated only with one type of VaD-multiple cortical infarctions and there are several other additional subtypes each aspecting a characteristic pattern of deficits[17]. Its prevalence in autopsy studies has been related to cortical and/or subcortical infarcts, focal, multiple or diffuse. They often involve strategically important brain areas, thalamus, frontobasal/limbic systems[18], white matter lesions and less often large brain areas. It is now known that even after a single infarction when located in a strategically important area in the brain can give rise to deficits in multiple areas of congnitive function[19]. The angular gyrus syndrome follows an infarction in the inferior parietal lobule and is characterized by aphasia, alexia, agraphia, Gerstman syndrome and constructional disturbances[20,21] and has a strong resemblance to the focal temporoparietal symptom pattern seen in AD. Other recognized strategic areas in the brain are genu of the internal capsule, thalamus, caudate, globus pallidus[19], basal forebrain and hippocampus. Strategic infarctions have unique features that reflect the specific brain region affected.

The LADIS Study demonstrated that lacunar infarcts in the putamen and globus pallidus affected memory, those in the thalamus are more likely to affect several cognitive domains and lacunar infarcts in the caudate, internal capsule and lobar white matter did not have any significant effects[22]. The penetrating arterioles and lenticulo-striate arteries supplying the deeper structures the basal ganglia and white matter are susceptible to arteriosclerotic injuries giving rise to lacunar infarctions and it has been shown that multiple lacunar infarctions can give rise to full dementia[19]. Subcortical infarctions have been shown to increase the risk of dementia by almost four times and reduce cognitive function and interact with Alzheimer's disease to worsen working memory[23]. Patients with high risk of dementia had cortical microinfarcts and to a lesser degree periventricular demyelination which contributed to the cognitive decline[24].

Several studies have shown increased white matter hyperintensities (WMH). WMH are associated with cognitive impairment even in the absence of dementia[25,26]. Imaging studies of white matter disease has raised interest in the role of white matter lesions in VaD. Leukoaraiosis meaning, 'rarefaction of white matter' can be subdivided into deep white matter and periventicular white matter lesions, and both have different pathogenesis and which is more damaging to cognition is unclear. Several published data however favour the periventricular lesions. In the Rotterdam Study periventricular lesions were correlated with rapid decline[27]. The PROGRESS trial further strengthened this notion that severe leukoaraiosis portends rapid progression. The study demonstrated that those with no leukoaraiosis at study entry was associated with 4% dementia or severe cognitive impairment after a four year follow-up. Whereas 30% of those with severe leukoaraiosis at study entry declined to this level[28].

MRI and autopsy studies have shown chronic hypoxia in areas of leukoaraiosis and some suggestion the hypoxia may be less pronounced in the periventicular white matter lesions and these are associated with ependymal loss [29] suggesting WMH may rise from a vascular cause[30]. Cardiovascular risk factors have an impact on vascular function and has been associated with increased WMH[18]. It appears that those factors leading to leukoaraiosis are specific to the cerebral vessels and that leukoaraiosis predicts stroke but does not predict other vascular events[31]. Endothelial dysfunction has been implicated as mechanism underlying leukoaraiosis[30]. Leukoaraiosis on CT is seen as diffuse hypodense areas in the white matter surrounding the ventricles (Fig 16.1). On MRI on the T2 images they appear as high signal intensities. (Fig.16.2 a and b.)

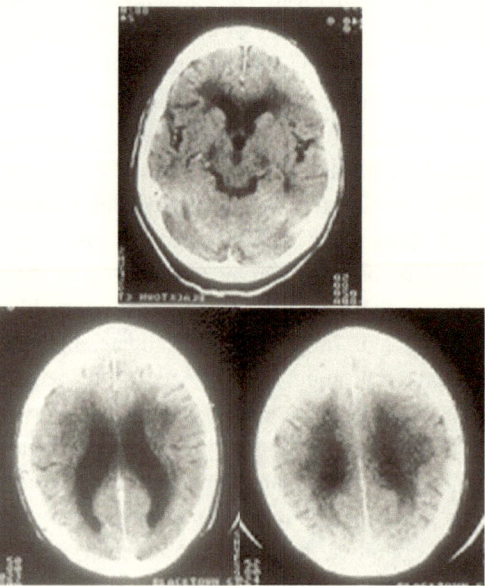

Fig 16.1. CT scan in leukoaraiosis shows severe low density areas around
the frontal and surrounding the lateral ventricles

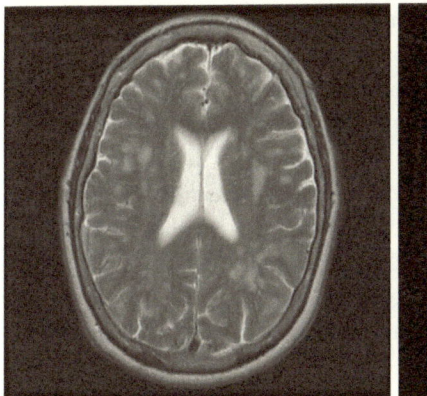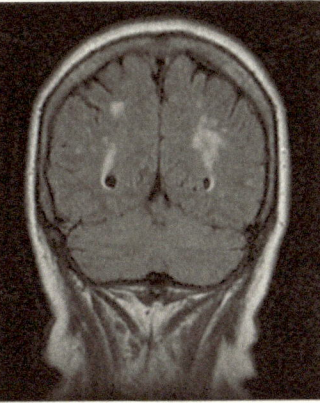

Fig.16.2. T2—weighted axial MRI scan above shows multifocal deep white matter lesions and below—proton-density coronal MRI shows periventricular lesions adjacent to the ventricles and deep white matter lesions distinctly away from the ventricles.

Discussion

Lacunar state and Binswanger's disease are two types of VaD associated with small vessel disease. Binswanger's disease is the result of multiple cumulative occlusions of the deep penetrating arterioles supplying the white matter. Both produce dementia syndrome with characteristic subcortical dementia including slowing of information processing, impaired memory and poor sustained attention, parkinsonism with prominent gait disturbances in conjunction with pyramidal tract signs, dysarthria, pseudobulbar affect, incontinence are frequent motor manifestations of VaD with small vessel disease[32]. Binswanger's disease has a wide spectrum of presentation, including dementia, a gait disorder not uncommonly seizures. BD is characterized by hypertension, discrete strokes, acute with or without recovery, subacute deficits, plateau periods and insidious memory loss leading to dementia[33,34].

Gorelick[35] considered the risks factors as 'putative' or 'tentative' for the reasons there has been no general consensus about the risk factors for VaD and the likely explanation for this are the studies of different populations using disparate methods. The potential risk factors being demographic, atherogenic, genetic and stroke—related factors[35]. Cerebral autosomal dominant arteriopathy with subcortical infarctions and leucoencephalopathies (CADASIL) is linked to chromosome 19. It causes subcortical lacunar infarction and dementia in over 80% of cases. The age of onset is in the forties with progression or stepwise course. Manifestations of the disorder include migraine, with aura, pseudo-bulbar features, mood disorders and dementia[36].

Silent cerebral infarcts that are strategically placed in the deep frontal lobe and thalamus may prove significant in the pathogenesis of dementia associated with stroke[35] Although the prevalence ranges from 12.9 percent[37] to 38 percent[38] the true prevalence in the general population is not known. Vascular lesions involving the frontal lobe may mimic AD with frontal involvement and the frontal variant of frontotemporal dementia (FTD). AD patients usually present with cognitive rather than social breakdown as well as personality change. In FTD the latter occur early with close similarities to the vascular frontal syndromes However the onset is insidious with degenerative dementias and is progressive[39].

An important overlap between AD and vascular disorder exists. Vascular lesions in AD include multicortical microinfarcts, subcortical lacunes, white matter lesions, small haemorrhages, cortico-subcortical infarcts, mixed type dementia, multiple large or hemispherics infarcts are frequent[18] The coincidence of AD and vascular disorders giving rise to a mixed dementia accounts for an approximately 15-19% of all dementia cases.

Diagnosis

The accuracy of diagnosis of VaD is found wanting because of limitations of assessment scales available. Most criteria used in the diagnosis of dementia emphasize memory impairment[40], which is not a common finding in cognitive impairment with VaD. Cognition assessed by the Mini-Mental State examination (MMSE) is inadequate as it insensitive to several domains commonly compromised in VaD. Several groups have proposed criteria for its diagnosis[41], but these criteria have been proposed for different purposes. Wetterling et al[42] compared the different diagnostic criteria for VaD and dicussed their limitations. The Hachinski Ischaemic scale is used in the diagnosis of VaD although it it more widely used for research purposes. Furthermore it has poor interrater reliability, is based on the concept that VaD is caused by multi-infarction and does not include neuro-imaging[40]. The DSM-IV criteria published by the American Psychiatric Association [44] has not been validated. The International Classification of Disease (ICD-10) produced by the World Health Organisation[44] subclassifies it into multi-infarction dementia, subcortical vascular dementia, vascular dementia of acute onset and mixed forms or unspecified types.

The National Instuitute of Neurological Disorders and Stroke and expert panel (NINDS-AIREN) (1993) used for a diagnosis of probable VaD requires the presence of (a) dementia (b) cerebrovascular disease and (c) a relation between the two (such as onset of dementia within three months of a stroke). The NINDS-AIREN and the criteria for the diagnosis proposed by the State of California Alzheimer's Disease Diagnostic and Treatment Centers[41] incorporate neuroimaging technology, comprehensive neuropsychological parameters and brain necropsy findings to help to elucidate vascular mechanisms that may cause cognitive impairment. These criteria has been criticised for being over inclusive and overlapping and have not been validated[35]. According to Roman[46] the diagnosis of poststroke VaD is fortright as most cases fulfill the NINDS-AREN criteria that is, there is acute onset of dementia, relevant cerebrovascular lesions demonstrated by neuroimaging and a time relationship between stroke and cognitive loss.

A high percentage of patients become demented following a stroke and about two-thirds are said to be aphasic[46]. The type of aphasia will depend on the location of the lesion. The true incidence in this category is not known, since most studies have excluded patients with severe aphasia because of the difficulties in testing them adequately[46]. The presence of dementia was assessed by using the functional criterion[46]. Censori et al[46] considered only those aphasic patients showing marked functional impairment that could not be explained by their communication deficits or hemiparesis.

Jorm and Korten[47] studied the feasibility of measuring cognitive decline in the elderly directly from informants. They developed a standardized interview to measure decline in both intelligence and memory of an elderly person's performance and ten years earlier. They found this to be a valid measure of cognitive decline and had less contamination with pre-morbid ability than the MMSE. The use of informants had also been suggested by Henderson and Huppert[48] for the diagnosis of early dementia because they are better informed as to the patient's performance. Other workers found informant reports have little validity as to memory functioning in normal elderly. Until guidelines for a reliable criteria are established the clinician should assess the aphasic patient and suspect dementia in a global way and not just in one aspect of the patient's symptomatology[49].

Management

Prevention—The risk factors should be looked for and modified. The main risk factors are listed in Table 16.1. The main risk factors are hypertension, diabetes, history of cardiovascular disease, cigarette smoking, sleep apnoea and more recently chronic infection and an elevated C-Reactive protein have been identified especially in diabetes[50]. VaD incidence can be decreased with primary and secondary prevention[51].

Treatment—Cholinesterase deficits have been demonstrated in VaD (independent of any concomitant AD pathology) including reduced choline acetyltransferase in the brain and low acetylcholine in cerebrospinal fluid[45]. Symptomatic cholinergic treatment has shown promise in AD with VaD and in probable VaD [51].

Table 16.1. Risk factors—and treatment

1. hypertension, diabetes—anti hypertensives

2. atrial fibrillation-anticoagulant

3. carotid artery disease—surgery

4. vasculitis-steroids, immunosuppressive drugs

5. cerebral hypoperfusion secondary to hyperviscosity syndrome—surgery

6. hereditary vascular dementia-

7. genetic counselling

CLINICAL RELEVANCE—
VASCULAR COGNITIVE IMPAIRMENT/VASCULAR DEMENTIA

* The term vascular cognitive impairment (VCI) had been proposed in place of vascular dementia (VaD) as it includes a wide range of cognitive decline ranging from mild deficits in one or more cognitive domains to a broad dementia-like syndrome[6]

* It ia a heterogenous disorder and the pathology may include the following: large infarcts, multiple lacunar infarcts, single infarcts in strategic locations, white matter lesions (leucoaraiosis) and low flow states.

* Symptoms may include functional impairment rather than memory early in the disease, prominent gait disturbances and falls, urinary incontinence and slowing of information processing.

* The main risk factors are hypertension, diabetes, history of cardiovascular disease, cigarette smoking and sleep apnoea and more recently reports of chronic infection and an elevated C-Reactive protein especially in diabetics.

* Approximately one-third of stroke survivors over the age of 75 years suffer from dementia.

* The diagnosis of poststroke VaD is fortright as most cases fulfill the NINDS-AREN criteria that is, there is acute onset of dementia, relevant cerebrovascular lesions demonstrated by neuroimaging and a time relationship between stroke and cognitive loss[46].

* Individuals with white matter disease may show cognitive slowing and gait disturbances but again CT and MRI may show white matter changes in normal older individuals.

* An important overlap between AD and vascular disease exists and there is a renewed interest whether vascular changes or brain changes are risk factors for AD.

* The occurrence of AD and vascular disorders giving rise to a mixed dementia accounts for about 15-20% of all dementia cases.

* Symptomatic cholinergic treatment has shown promise in AD with VaD and in probable VaD[51].

REFERENCES

1. Hachinski VC, Lassen NA, Marshall J. Multi-infarct dementia—a case of mental deterioration in the elderly. *Lancet* 1974; ii: 207-209.-
2. Scheinberg P. Dementia due to vascular disease-A multifactorial disorder. *Stroke* 1988; 19: 1291-1299.
3. Lodder J. Poststroke cognition and fight against the hard problem Editorial. *Stroke* 2007; 38: 7-8.
4. Hennerici MG. What are the mechanisms for post stroke dementia? *The Lancet Neurology* 2009; 8(11): 973-975.
5. Cherubini A, Senin U. Elderly stroke patient at risk for dementia: In search of a profile. Editorial Comment. *Stroke* 2003; 34: 2245.
6. Erkinjuntti T, Gauthier S. The concept of vascular cognitive impairment. *Front Neurol Neurosci* 2009; 24:79-85 (abstract).
7. Zhu Li, Fratiglioni L, Guo Z et al. Association of stroke with dementia, cognitive impairment and functional disability in the very old: a population based study. *Stroke* 1998: 29: 2094-2099.
8. Skoog I, Nilsson L, Palmertz B et al. A population based study of dementia in 85 year olds. *N Engl J Med* 1993; 328: 153-158.
9. Jorm AF, Korten AE, Henderson AS. The prevalence of dementia: a quantitative fintegration of the literature. *Acta Psychiatr Scand* 1987;76: 465-478.
10. Rocca WA. The prevalence of vascular dementia in Europe-facts and fragments from 1980-1990 studies. *Ann Neurol* 1991; 30: 817-824.
11. McKeith IG, Perry RH, Fairbain AF et al. Operational criteria for senile dementia of Lewy body type. *Psychol Med* 1992; 22: 911-922.
12. Tatemichi TK, Paik M, Bagiella E et al. Risk of dementia after stroke in a hospitalized cohort: results of a longitudinal study. *Neurology* 1994; 44: 1885-1892.
13. Pohjasvaara T, Erkinjunti T, Ylikoski R et al. Clinical determinants of poststroke dementia. *Stroke* 1998: 29:75-81.
14. Rocca WA, Bonaiuto S, Lippi A et al. Prevalence of clinically diagnosed Alzheimer's disease and other dementing disorders: a door—to-door survey. in Appignario Macerata Province, Italy. *Neurology* 1990; 40: 626-531.
15. Magnusson H. Mental health of octogenarians in Iceland. An epidemiological study. *Acta Psychiatr Scand* (suppl) 1989; 79: 1-112.
16. Gorelick PB. Stroke prevention. *Arch Neurol* 1995; 52: 347-354.
17. McPherson SE, Cummings JL. Neuropsychological aspects of vascular dementia. *Brain-Cogn* 1996; 31:269-82.
18. Jellinger KA. Pathology and pathophysiology of vascular cognitive impairment. A critical update. *Panminerva Med* 2004; 46(4): 217-26 (abstract).

19. Scott TM, Folstein MF. Cognition and neuropsychology in Cerebrovascular Disease and Dementia. Ed. Edmond Chiu, Lars Gustafson, David Ames and Marshal F Folstein. Martin Dunitz,2001. Chap.13 pp131-134.

20. Cummings JL, Benson DF. Dementia: a clinical approach Butterworth—Heinemann, Boston.1992.

21. Nagaratnam N, Phan TA, Barnett C, Ibrahim N. Angular gyrus-like syndrome mimicking depressive pseudo-dementia. *J Psychiatr Neurosci* 2002; 27(5): 364-368.

22. Benisty S, Gouw AA, Porcher R et al. On behalf of the LADIS Study group: Location of lacunar infarcts correlates with cognition in a sample of non-disabled subjects with age-related white matter changes: the LADIS study. J *Neurol Neurosurg Psychiatry* 2009; 80: 478-483.

23. Schneider JA, Boyle PA, Arvanitakis Z et al. Subcortical infarcts, Alzheimer's disease, pathology and memory function in older persons. *Ann Neurol* 2007; 62: 59-66.

24. Kovari E, Gold G, Herrmann FR et al. Cortical microinfarcts and demyelination affect cognition in cases at high risk for dementia. *Neurology* 2007; 68: 927-931.

25. Paul RH, Haque O, Gunstad J et al. Subcortical hyperintensities impact cognitive function among a select subset of healthy elderly. *Arch Clin Neuropsychol* 2005; 20: 697-704.

26. Gunning-Dixon PM, Raz N. Neuroanatomic correlates of selected executive functions in middle-aged and older adults. *Neuropsychologia* 2003; 41: 1929-1941.

27. van Dijk EJ, Prins ND, Vrooman HA et al. Progression of cerebral small vessel disease in relation to risk factors and cognitive consequences: Rotterdam Scan Study. *Stroke* 2008; 39: 2712-2710.

28. Dufouil C, Godin O, Chalmers J et al. for the Progress MRI Substudy Investigators. Severe cerebral white matter hyperintensities predict severe cognitive decline in patients with cerebrovascular disease history. *Stroke* 2009; 40: 2219-2221.

29. Bowler JV, Gorelick PB. Advances in vascular cognition impairment—2006. *Stroke* 2007; 38: 41-244.

30. Hoth KF, Tate DF, Poppas A et al. Endothelial function and white matter hyperintensities in older adults with cardiovascular disease. *Stroke* 2007; 38: 308-312.

31. Buyck J-F, Dufouil C, Mazoyer B. et al. Cerebral white matter lesions are associated with risk of stroke but not with other vascular events:the 3-City Dijon study. *Stroke* 2009; 40: 2327-2331.

32. Cummings JL. Vascular subcortical dementias. clinical apects. *Dementia* 1994; 5: 177-180.

33. Caplan LR, Schene WC. Clinical features subcortical arteriosclerotic encephalopathy (Binswanger's Disease). *Neurology* 1979; 28: 1206-1218.

34. Nagaratnam N, Beves A, Nagaratnam S. Binswanger's disease presenting as progressive speech disorder with CT and MRI findings. *Eur J Int Med* 1994; 5: 321-323.

35. Gorelick PB. Status of risk factors for dementia associated with stroke. *Stroke* 1997; 28: 459-463.

36. Chabriat H, Vaheda K, Iba-Zizen MT et al. Spectrum of CADASIL; a study of seven families. *Lancet* 1995; 346: 934-939.

37. Shinkawa A, Ueda K, Kiyohara Y et al. Silent cerebral infarction in a community-based autopsy series in Japan. *Stroke* 1995; 26: 380-385.

38. Ricci S, Celani MG, La Rosa F et al. Silent brain infarction in patients with first-ever stroke: a community based study in Umbera, Italy. *Stroke* 1993; 24: 647-651.

39. Nagaratnam N, Bou-Haidar P, Leung H. Confused and disturbed behaviour in the elderly following silent frontal lobe infarction. *Amer J Alz Dis* 2003 18; 333-339.

40. Hachinski VC, Illif LD, ilhka E et al. Cerebral blood flow in dementia. *Arch Neurol* 1975; 32: 632-637.

41. Chui HC, Victoroff J, Margolin D et al, Criteria for the diagnosis of ischaemic vascular dementia proposed by the state of California Alzheimer's Disease Diagnostic and Treatment Centers. *Neurology* 1992; 42: 473-480.

42. Wetterling T, Kanitz RD, Borgis JK. Comparison of different diagnostic criteria for vascular dementia (ADDTC, DSM-IV, ICD-10, NINDS-AIREN). *Stroke* 1996; 21; 30-35.

43. American Psychiatric Association. Diagnostic and Statistical Manual of Mental Disorders (4th ed) (DSM-IV). Washington DC. American Psychiatric Association. 1994.

44. World Health Organisation. The ICD-10 Classification of Mental and Behavioural Disorders. Clinical description and diagnostic guidelines. Geneva. Switzerland. World Health Organisation.199250-51.

45. Roman GC. Facts, myths and controversies in vascular dementia. *J Neurosci Sci* 2004; 226: 49-52(abstract).

46. Censori B, Manara O, Agostinis C et al. Dementia after first stroke. *Stroke* 1996; 27: 1205-1210.

47. Jorm AF, Korten AE. Assessment of cognitive decline in the elderly by informant. interview. *Br J Psychiatry* 1988; 152: 209-215.

48. AS, Huppet FA. The problem of mild dementia. *Psychol Med* 1984; 14: 5-11.

49. Nagaratnam N, O'Neill C. Dementia in the severely aphasic: global aphasia without hemiparesis-a stroke subtype simulating dementia. *Amer J Alz Dis* 1999, 14: 74-78.

50. Roman GC. Vascular dementia prevention: a risk analysis. *Cerebrovasc Dis* 2005; 20 Suppl 2: 91-100 (abstract).

51. Erkinjuntti T. Diagnosis and management of vascular cognitive impairment and dementia. *J Neurol Transm Suppl* 2002;(63): 91-109(abstract).

17

STROKE PROCLIVITY FOR

FALLS IN THE ELDERLY

Introduction

Falls are a growing concern in the elderly population. Falls in the elderly stroke patient can be attributed to several factors with an enormous amount of individual risk factors. It is imperative for those treating the elderly stroke victims to have a clear understanding of the changes associated with stroke. Neurological, physical and psychological changes occur not only with stroke but also with ageing.

Incidence prevalence and epidemiology

The risk of falls is especially high among stroke patients[1,2]. Forster and Young[3] reported that 73% of the participants in their study fell in the first 6 months after the stroke, a significant increase from the annual incidence of 30% in community dwelling elderly[4]. Falling is one of the most important complications among stroke patients in rehabilitation[5,6]. Between 14% and 65% of stroke survivors experience falls while in hospital[5,7,8]. Women are more likely to fall than men but some studies have shown no important gender differences[1]. Falls in general are associated with considerable mortality and morbidity and cause three types of morbidity namely, injury, restrictions of mobility and walking and psychological distress[9]. 80-90% of injuries are caused by falls in various forms of geriatric care[10,11].

Pathophysiology

There is no widely accepted classification of falls[12]. Tinetti et al[13] examined and subdivided falls into,1. situational, identified as acute host-related risk taking activities and 2. predisposing risk factors such as medical, sensory, neurological, musculoskeletal and medicine. Incidence of strokes increases with age. Falls result from a single or combination of environmental and medical factors that interact with physiological age—related changes.

218

The efficiency of the physiological systems for postural control diminishes with age. Postural stability or balance is maintained by continued adjustments to sensory outputs—visual, vestibular and somatosensory[14] which tend to diminish with age. They play an important role in causing falls in the elderly. Visual acuity, auditory function and tactile sensation are blunted with ageing. Impaired vision, peripheral vision, depth perception can lead to impaired ability to cope with environmental demands, loss of balance and falls[15]. Impaired sense of vibration in the legs as well as impaired perception increases postural sway[16]. Postural instability or sway is due to decreased sensory input slowing down of the motor responses and weakness of support[17]. In old age the integrated sensory inputs[18] together with the slower rate of central processing[19,20] lead to difficulties in co-ordination of reflexes and voluntary movements in postural control.

In stroke changes in stability, balance, muscle strength and co-morbidities are precipitating factors for falls. Studies have shown that postural sway, cognitive and behavioural deficits and moderate to severe disability on admission were common in patients who fall[5]. Components of the sensori-motor system also contribute to balance problems. Among fallers vertigo and antihypertensive drugs intake are predictors of falls[21]. Stroke and vascular disease of the labyrinth are leading causes of central vestibular disturbances[21]. Spasticity which results from an upper motor neurone syndrome may negatively affect mobility, balance and gait increasing the risk of falls and fractures[22].

Rehabilitation has been an important component in stroke care. There is a high rate of falls during rehabilitation. Characteristically associated with falls in the rehabilitation hospital included advanced age (>50 years), diagnosis of stroke or lower limb amputation compared to patients with trauma[1]. Risk factors associated with falls in stroke patients have been studied in acute care and rehabilitation settings[5,23,24]. Wheelchair falls were attributed to leaning or reaching out from chairs and to transfers from wheel chairs[1]. Rapport et al[23] found that impulsive behaviour related to right hemispheric stroke increased fall risk. Fig.17.1.

Discussion

In the elderly stroke patient falls are an accumulated effect of multiple risk factors. Changes in stability, muscle strength and coordination are predisposing factors for falls in stroke patients. Affected by other deconditioning effects of prolonged bed rest such as decreased cardiac output and decline in blood volume[25]. Stroke specific impairments such as neglect or inattention may contribute to falls risk[26]. Some stroke types such as lesions in the thalamus are known to cause disturbance in sitting and standing balance[27,28]. Thalamic astasia and unilateral asterexis occurring with thalamic lesions have been associated with disordered postural tone. Small infarcts strategically placed are capable of causing deficits the nature of which will depend on the location and distribution of the lesion.

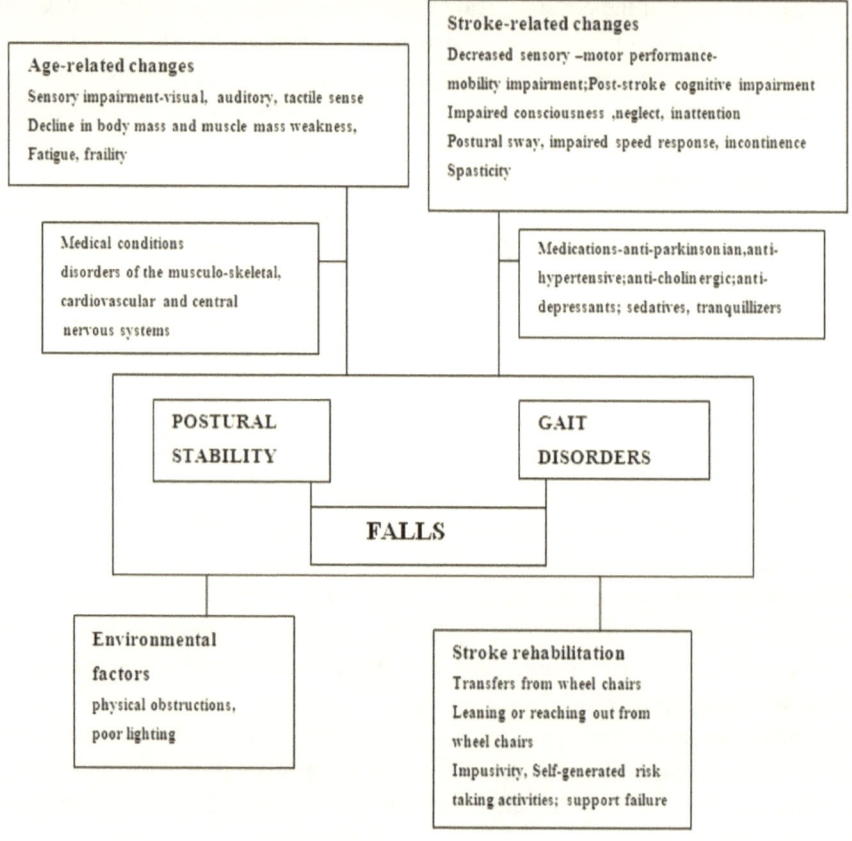

Fig.17.1 Pathophysiology of falls in stroke
Information sources: see text

The physical complications of falls are fractures which amounts to about 50% and their complications that can lead todeath in a significant number of cases[29]. Hip fracture constitute a leading cause of hospital admissions and prolonged stay among the elderly. Furthermore 90% of hip fractures are caused by a fall and 1% of the falls result in hip fracture[30].

A post-fall syndrome has been recognized which combines backward disequilibrium in sitting and standing positions and gait modifications[31]. Psychological distress has been consistently mentioned as the main consequence associated with falls. Psychomotor disadaptation syndrome (PDS) is characterised by loss of independence, loss of self confidence, restrictions in mobility and activity due to fear of falling, social withdrawal and risk of institutionalization[32]. Fear of falling has been identified in 50-60% of reported fallers[33]. Schmid and Rittman[34] studied the perceived consequence of post stroke falls. They found three primary consequences of poststroke falls namely activity and participation limitation, increased dependence and the development of fear of falling.

One of the main findings of high rate of falls during rehabilitation is falling from wheel chair and this has been attributed too improper techniques, wheel chair in poor repair and to host related activities[21]. In about 85% of the patients who fall exhibit risk taking activity during stroke rehabilitation and this is related to post stroke cognitive impairment[21].

Evaluation and Management

Evaluation of mobillty/gait and balance play an important part of a comprehensive assessment. Useful information as to the level of dysfunction can be obtained from simple clinical tests such as the 'Timed Up and Go' test[35] and the 'One-Leg balance[36]. These tests have indicated a strong correlation with a history of falls. Furthermore the functional balance measures are quantifiable and compare well with the ability of the elderly to ambulate safely[37].

In spite of the evidence for the different and effective interventions in reducing falls in the elderly in general there is limited evidence in relation to stroke survivors[26]. It is important to identify factors associated with falls that are amenable to correction and to treat the remediable pathology. If a single cause is not identified but many potential processes are found, management should be directed toward correcting these factors. The medications should be reviewed. Balance performance can be improved by balance training, namely muscle strength exercises[38], specific balance exercises, for example walking and co-ordination exercises, dancing and tai chi movements, and using sensory input manipulation[39]. Physiotherapy can improve mobility. In those with vestibular defects vestibular rehabilitation therapies have been beneficial. Environment hazards have to be eliminated and there may be a need for institutional placement (Table 17.1).

A program of secondary prevention of falls should be adhered to. Specific interventions should be instituted based on individual's risk factors, by (i) changes in life style namely to cease smoking, moderate consumption of alcohol and to increase physical activity and (ii) reviewing medications (iii) assessing for sensory deficits-visual defects, gait and balance, and muscle weakness and (iv) Vitamin D supplementation[40].

In a review, Batchelor et al[26] reported that vitamin D supplementation reduced falls in female stroke survivors in the institutional setting. The possibility of extending this preventive vitamin D therapy to all stroke survivors needs further study[26]. The explanation for the effectiveness of vitamin D is attributed to the action of vitamin D on muscle and central nervous system function[40]. Vitamin D with or without calcium contributed to muscle strength and improves postural balance and navigation abilities and decreased risk of falls[40].

Table 17. 1 Management of falls

Identify correctable factors and treat

Review medications

Improve balance performances

    i. improve muscle strength

    ii. institute specific balance exercises

    iii. use sensory input manipulation

    iv. vestibular rehabilitation therapies
       where indicated

Physiotherapy to improve mobility

Eliminate environmental hazards

Determine need for placement

Institute secondary prevention of falls

Use of hip protectors

```
┌─────────────────────────────────────────────┐
│            CLINICAL RELEVANCE—              │
│  STROKE PROCLIVITY FOR FALLS IN THE ELDERLY  │
└─────────────────────────────────────────────┘
```

* The risk of falls is especially high in stroke patients and is an important complication among stroke patients in rehabilitation.
* Between 14% and 65% of stroke survivors experience falls while in hospital.
* In the elderly stroke patient falls are an accumulated effect of multiple risk factors.
* One of the main findings of high rate of falls during rehabilitation is falling from wheel chair attributed too improper techniques, wheel chair in poor repair and to host related activities.
* In about 85% of the patients who fall exhibit risk taking activity during stroke rehabilitation and this is related to post stroke cognitive impairment.
* Consequences of falls post-stroke are limitation of participation and activity, fear of falling and increased dependence.
* It is important to identify factors associated with falls that are amenable to correction and to treat the remediable pathology.
* Vitamin D supplementation contributes to improved muscle strength and reduced risk of falls[40].

REFERENCES

1. Vlahov D, Myers AH, Al-Ibrahim MS. Epidemiology of falls among patients in a rehabilitation hospital. *Arch Phys Med Rehabil* 1990; 71: 8-12.

2. DeVicenzo DK, Watkins S. Accidental falls in a rehabilitation center. *Rehabil Nurs* 1987; 12: 248-252.

3. Forster A, Young J. Incidence and consequence of falls due to stroke. A systemic inquiry. *Brit. Med J* 1995; 311: 83-88.

4. Tinetti ME, Speechley M, Ginter SF. Risk factors for falls among elderly persons living in the community. *New Eng J Med* 1988, 319: 1701

5. Nyberg L, Gustafson Y. Patient falls in stroke rehabilitation. *Stroke* 1995; 26: 838-842.

6. Dromerick A, Reding M. Medical and neurological complications during stroke inpatients rehabilitation. *Stroke* 1994; 25: 358-361.

7. Davenport RJ, Dennis MS., Wellwood I, Warlow CP. Complications of acute stroke *Stroke*; 1996;27:415-420.

8. Teasell R, McRae M, Foley N, Bhardwaj A. AThe incidence and consequences of falls in stroke patients during in patient rehabilitation: Factors associated with high risk. *Arch Phys Med Rehabil.* 2002; 83: 329-333.

9. Cwikel F, Fried AV. The social epidemiology of falls among community dwelling elderly: guidelines for prevention. *Disability and Rehabilitation.*1992; 14: 113-121.

10. Lee RG. Health safety in hospitals. *Med Sci Law* 1979; 19: 89-103.

11. Uden G. Inpatients accidents in hospitals. *J Am Geriat Soc.* 1985; 33: 833-841.

12. Blake AJ, Morgan K, Bendall MJ et al. Falls by elderly people at home: prevalence and associated factors. *Age and Aging* 1988; 17; 365-372.

13. Tinetti M, Doucette JT, Clous EB. The contribution of predisposing situational risk Factors to serious fall injuries. *J Am Geriatr Soc.* 1995; 43: 1207-1213.

14. Lee D, Lishman R. Vision in movement and balance. New Sci 1975; 9: 59-61

15. Gerson LW, Jarjoura D, McCord G. Risk of imbalance in elderly people with impaired hearing or vision. *Age and Ageing* 1989; 18: 31-34.

16. Brockelhurst JC, Robertson D, James-Groin P. Clinical correlates of sway in old age-sensory modalities. *Age Aging,* 1982; 11: 1-10.

17. Baloh RW, Fife TD, Zwerling L et al. Comparison of static and dynamic posturography in young and older normal people. *J Am Geriatr Soc.* 1994; 42: 404-416.

18. Manchester D, Woollacott M, Zoderbauer-Hylton N, Marino O. Visual, vestibular and somato-sensory contributions to balance control in older adults. *J Gerontol* 1989; 44:M118-M127.

19. Stelmach GE, Worringham CJ. Sensation for deficits related to postural stability implications for falling in the elderly. *Clin Geriatr Med.* 1984; 1: 679-694.

20. Woollacott M, Shunway-Cook SA, Nashner L. Aging and postural control. Changes in sensory organization in muscular co-ordination. *Int J Aging Hum Dev* 1986; 23: 97-114.
21. Aizen E, Shugaev I, Lenger R. Risk factors and characteristic falls during inpatient rehabilitation of elderlty patients *Arch Geront Geriatrics* 2007; 44: 1-12.
22. Esquenazi A. Falls and fractures in older poststroke patients wuth spasticity consequences and drug treatment considerations. *Clin Geriatrics* 2004; 12. *http://www.clinicalgeriatrics.com/article/3430* accessed 28/02/2010
23. Rapport IJ, Webster JS, Flemming KL. et al. Predictors of falls among right hemispheric stroke patients in the rehabilitation setting. *Arch Phys Med Rehabil* 1993; 74: 621-626.
24. Byers V, Arrington ME Finstuen K. Predictive risk factors associated with stroke patient falls in acute care settings *J Neurosci Nurs* 1990; 22: 147-154.
25. Fortney SM, Turner C, Steinmann L et al. Blood volume responses of men and women to bed rest. *J Clin Pharmacol* 1994; 34: 434-439.
26. Batchelor F, Hill K, Mackintosh S, Said C. What works in falls prevention after stroke? Asystematic review and meta-analysis. *Stroke* 2010; 41: 1715-1722.
27. Masdeu JC, Gorelick PB. Thalamic astasia: Instability to stand after unilateral thalamic lesions. *Ann Neurol* 1988; 223: 596-603.
28. Nagaratnam N, Leung H, Bou-Haider P. Lacunar stroke proclivity for falls. *Int J Clin Pract* 2004; 58: 83-86.
29. Gibson MJ, Andres K, Isaacs B et al. Prevention of falls in later life. *Danish Medical Bulletin.* 1987; 49 Supp 4):1-24.
30. Nevitt MC, Cummings SR, Hudes ES. Risk factor for injurious falls: a prospective study. *J Gerontol.*1991; 46: M164-M170.1707
31. Manckoundia P, Gerbault N, Mourey F et al. Multidisciplinary management in geriatric day-hospital is beneficial for elderly fallers: A prospective study of 28 cases *Arch Geront Geriatr,.* 2007; 44: 61-70
32. Pfitzenmeyer P, Mourey F, Tavernier B, Camus A. Psychomotor disadaptation syndrome. *Arch Gerontol Geriatr* 1999; 28: 217-225.
33. Powell LE, Myers AM. The Activities-Specific Balance Confidence (ABC) Scale. J Gerontl. 1995; 50A: M28-M34
34. Schmid AA, Rittman H. Consequences of poststroke falls activity limitation, increased dependence and development of fear of falling. *Am J Occup Therapy* 2009. *http://www.thefreelibrary.com/Consequences+of+poststroke+falls+activity+limitation_i . . . 28/02/2010*
35. Podsladdo D, Richardson S. The timed "Up and Go", a test of basic functional mobility in frail elderly persons. *J Am Geriatr Soc* 1991; 39:142-8
36. Vellas BJ, Wayne SJ, Romero L et al. One leg balance is an important predictor of injurious falls in older persons. *J Am Geriatr Soc* 1997; 45: 735-8.
37. Fuller GF. Falls in the elderly. *Am Fam Physician* 2000; 81: 2159-68,2173-4.

38. Lord S, Ward J, Williams P Anstey K. An epidemiological study of falls in older community-dwellling women. The Randwick falls and fractures study. *Aust J Public Health* 1993; 17: 240-245.

39. Hu MH, Woollacott MH. Multisensory training of standing balance in older adults.I. Postural stability and one leg stance balance. *J Gerontol* 1994; 49: M52-M61.

40. Annweiler C, Montero-Odass M, Schott AM et al. Fall prevention and vitamin D in elderly: an overview of the key role of non-bone effects . *J Neuroeng Rehabil* 2010;7:50 doi:10.1186/1743-0003-50

18

POST-STROKE SEIZURES

IN THE ELDERLY

Introduction

In the elderly stroke is the common cause of seizures. Furthermore seizures are the most common neurological consequence of stroke. Approximately 10% of stroke patients experience seizures[1]. Seizures may be early or late complication of stroke and are the result of focal or generalized distrurbance of cerebral function which maybe due to various cerebral or systemic disorders. Seizures associated with stroke are categorized as occurring immediately before, immediately after (within 24 hours) or of early or late onset[2]. Early—onset seizures have a peak onset within the first day after the stroke and tend to be focal, motor brief and isolate[3]. Late-onset seizures have a peak onset within 6 to 12 months after the stroke[4]. About one third with early—onset seizures and one-half with late-onset seizures develop epilepsy[4]. In upto 28% of patients develop their first seizure several years later[5] .

Incidence prevalence and epidemiology

The average age of patients with poststroke seizures (PSS) is 55.4 years[6]. Epilepsy often develop for the first time in old age. The incidence of the first seizure is 52-59 per 100,000 in persons 40-59 years and this rises to 127 per 100,000 in the 60 years or more[7]. The active prevalence rate is approximately 1.5% among the 65 years and older. Seizures occur with a frequency of 10.6 and 8.5% in haemorrhagic and ischaemic stroke respectively and in subarachnoid haemorrhage it is 8.5% and the late onset occurs 3 times more often than the early onset [5].

Epilepsy (recurrent seizures) develops in 3% to 4% of the stroke patients and accounts for 30-40% of cases of epilepsy[8]. In a population based study of the incidence of epilepsy and unprovoked seizures for persons with identified etiology, cerebrovascular disease accounted for 35% in the age group 35-65 years and 67% in the elderly aged more than 65 years[7].

Pathophysiology

The elderly are more prone to develop seizures whether provoked by acute illness (provoked or acute symptomatic seizures) or without (unprovoked seizures) immediate cause[10]. The early—onset PSSs are considered to be provoked seizures and are said to be caused by acute metabolic and physiological derangements associated wth acute infarction[2] and once these derangements are reversed the seizures cease[3]. Whereas in haemorrhagic stroke the products of blood metabolism such as haemosiderin may cause a focal cerebral irritation leading to seizures and lobar haematomas are frequently accompanied by early—onset stroke—related seizures[5]. Seizures are more commonly associated with haemorrhagic rather than with ischaemic stroke[2]. The late—onset are considered to be unprovoked seizures that occur from partially injured brain giving rise to an epileptic focus[3]. Involvement of the cortex with stroke increases the risk of seizures. Deep—seated hemispheric or infratentorial lesions rarely produce seizure or epilepsy[3].

In a large series of patients with post stroke seizures 9% had status epilepticus[1]. Periodic lateralizing epileptiform discharges (PLEDS) have been commonly associated with cerebral infarction but also in other cerebral diseases such as encephalitis, tumour and demyelinating diseases[12]. PLEDs is characterized by repetitive spike or 'sharp' wave discharges focal or late changes over one hemisphere and occurring at fixed time intervals[12]. Patients with acute stroke and PLEDs are predisposed to the development of seizures[13]. The relationship between PLEDs, acute stroke and subsequent development of epilepsy is not clear. PLEDs have been considered as a part of status epilepticus[14].

Reperfusion syndrome or hyperperfusion syndrome is increase in the blood flow well above the metabolic demands of the brain. This can result in brain injury with fatal oedema or intracerebral haemorrhage. Rapid restoration of normal perfusion pressure can occur following thrombolytic therapy for acute ischaemic stroke. There is disruption of the blood brain barrier, cortical irritability and epileptic seizures. The cerebral reperfusion syndrome presents as ipsilateral severe headache, contralateral neurological deficits and seizure which maybe focal or generalized[15].

Evaluation of PSS

The differential diagnosis includes other causes of seizures and the conditions that can mimic seizures. The clinical presentation may not be typical, atypical seizure forms are seen especially in older people. They may present with symptoms of acute confusional state, behavioural changes or syncope[16]. Changes in the mental status in the elderly can be due to a number of causes and when the elderly patient presents with change in the mental state the diagnosis of epilepsy can be difficult. A common manifestation in the elderly is non-convulsing status epilepticus (NCSE). NCSE is now being increasingly recognized with the use of evolving EEG technology[17]. NCSE can occur in various settings, in patients with epilepsy or arising de novo or in the setting of acute or remote symptomatic conditions[17]. Many may not have a history of epilepsy[18] and there is often a long delay in the diagnosis[19]. There should be increased awareness and increased diagnostic suspicion. Elderly patients with unexplained episodes of confusion, disorientation, decreased consciouness and motor and sensory symptoms should be evaluated for seizures and an EEG video monitoring should be considered for such evaluation[13].

There are a number of conditions that can mimic seizures especially in the elderly. Transient ischaemic attacks (TIA) can be confused with seizures. Inhibiting seizures simulating TIA is seen in 7.1% of cases[5]. The 'shaking limb' TIAs which occur with carotid artery stenosis can be distinguished by its postural character, occurring on standing and not involving the facial muscles and cognition[20]. Others in the differential diagnosis include syncope, migraine, toxic metabolic diseases and narcolepsy.

Treatment

Monotherapy is the main goal of epileptic treatment and controls about two-thirds of the patients with epilepsy[16]. Generally there are no significant differences in the effectiveness of the anti-epileptic drugs (AEDs) if they are adequately used in relation to the type of seizure. The problems lie with the side-effects and interactions.

The newer drugs such as gabapantin, lamotrigine, oxcarbazepine, levetiracetam, tiagabine, topiramate appear to be better tolerated with regard to mood and cognitive effects[21] but are more expensive. The older drugs phenytoin, sodium valproate and carbamazepine are effective against partial seizures with or without secondary generalizations but are associated with substantial risk of osteoporosis.

With increasing age the pharmacokinetics and pharmacodynamics of the AEDs undergo alteration. Thus the mechanisms of the actions of the drugs should be taken into account as well as metabolic routes to minimize drug interactions. In the elderly the biological age is more important than the chronological age in terms of choice and usage of AEDs [22]. AEDs that cause cognitive impairment are best avoided. The main limitations for all these AEDs are those associated with sedation[16].

In selecting a drug for the elderly special consideration should be given to co-existing medical conditions[21]. For instance in patients with hepatic failure the first consideration in the choice of the drug should be an agent mainly excreted by the kidney and for one with renal failure an agent metabolised by the liver.

Carbamazepine, lamotrigine, sodium valproate and topiramate are the first line AEDs recommended[23]. There is a good correlation between the dose and plasma concentration for carbamazepine (plasma therapeutic range 20-50umol/l)[16]. The so-called therapeutic levels can cause problems especially in the elderly for these levels have been derived from a non-elderly population[21]. The doses that seem to be more appropriate are in the lower levels than the therapeutic ones and the clinician is best placed to decide[21]. The elderly are very susceptible to adverse effects and clear cut consideration should be given to the most appropriate AED minimizing its side effects and potential drug interactions. Most elderly people respond well to AEDs including low doses of AED[23]. Sometimes polytherapy may be necessary to control the seizures and when used it should be used judiciously. Elderly patients are often on multiple drugs and the use of AEDs that do not alter the metabolism of other drugs should be borne in mind. For example, neither gabapantin or levetiracetam alter the metabolism of other drugs or are altered by other drugs[13].

* In the elderly stroke is the common cause of seizures and may occur immediately before, immediately after (withn 24 hours), or of early or late onset.
* Seizures are more commonly associated with haemorrhagic rather than ischaemic stroke and involvement of the cortex increases the risk.
* In a large series of patients with post stroke seizures 9% had status epilepticus.
* Periodic lateralizing epileptiform discharges (PLEDS) have been commonly associated with cerebral infarction but also in other cerebral diseases such as encephalitis, tumour and demyelinating diseases[12].
* The cerebral reperfusion syndrome presents as ipsilateral severe headache, contralateral neurological deficits and seizure which maybe focal or generalized.
* NCSE can occur in various settings, in patients with epilepsy or arising de novo or in the setting of acute or remote symptomatic conditions[17].
* Monotherapy is the main goal of epileptic treatment and in the elderly special consideration should be given to co-existing medical conditions and side-effects.
* The newer drugs such as gabapantin, lamotrigine, oxcarbazepine, levetiracetam, tiagabine, topiramate appear to be better tolerated with regard to mood and cognitive effects.
* Carbamazepine, lamotrigine, sodium valproate, topiramate are the first line of AEDs recommended[16].
* The elderly are very susceptible to adverse effects and clear cut consideration should be given to the most appropriate AED minimizing its side effects and potential drug interactions.
* Most elderly people respond well to AEDs including low doses of AED.

REFERENCES

1. Silverman IE, Restrepo L, Mathews GC. Poststroke seizures. *Arch Neurol* 2002; 59: 195-201.
2. Kelly KM. Poststroke seizures and epilepsy: Clinical study and animal models. *Epilepsy Curr* 2002; 2(6): 873-877.
3. Asconape JJ, Penry JK. Poststroke seizures in the elderly. *Clin Geriatr Med* 1991;7(3): 483-92.
4. Olsen TS. Poststroke epilepsy. *Curr Athroscler Rep* 2001; 3: 340-4.
5. De Reuck JI. Management of stroke-related seizures. *Eur Neuro Dis.* 2008; 11: www: touchneurology.com/articles/management-stroke-related—seizures. 1/02/2010.
6. Teasell R, McRae M, Wiebe S. Poststroke seizures in stroke rehabilitation patients. *J Stroke Cerebrovas Dis* 2003; 8: 84-87.
7. Hauser WA. Epidemiology of seizures in the elderly. In Rowan AJ, Ramsay PE. Seizures and Epilepsy in the elderly. Butterworth-Heinmann 1997:7-20
8. Mohanraj R, Brodie MJ. Diagnosing refractory epilepsy: response to sequential treatment schedules. *Eur J Neurol* as quoted by Brodie and Kwan, 2005.
9. Hauser WA, Annegers JF, Kurland LT. Incidence of epilepsy and unprovoked seizures in Rochester. Minnesota:1935-1984. *Epilepsia* 1993; 34: 453-68 (Medline).
10. Brodie MJ, Kwan P. Epilepsy in elderly people. *BMJ* 2005; 331: 1317-22.
11. Velioglu S, Ozmenoglu M, Biz C, Alioglu Z. Status epilepticus after stroke. *Stroke* 2001;32:1169-1172.
12. Dan YF, Pan ABS, Lun SH. PLEDs: aetiology and association with EEG seizures. *Neurology (Asia)* 2004; 9: 107-108.
13. Holmes GL. The complex phenomenon of epilepsy in the elderly *http://www.medscape.com/viewarticle/49632* assessed on 11/14/2008.
14. Snodgrass SM, Kenji T, Cosimo AM. Clinical significance of PLED-relationship with status epilepticus. *J Clin Neurophysiol* 1989;6 (2):159:172 (abstract).
15. Elizawahry H, Hernandez-Frau PE, Behrouz R, Clark WM. Hyperperfusion in stroke. e Medicine Neurology. *http://emedicine.medscape.com/article/1162437-overview* Updated 24 June 2009. accessed 15/08/2010.
16. Myint PK, Staufenberg EFA, Sabanathan K. Poststroke seizure and poststroke epilepsy. *Postgrad med* 2006; 82: 568-572.
17. Waterhouse E. Status epilepticus in acute settings. *Epilepsy Curr* 2002; 2: 43-44.
18. Bottaro FJ, Reisin RC, Marinez OA et al. Nonconvulsive status epilepticus (NSCE) in the elderly population: a case—control study. Program and abstracts of the American Epilepsy Society 58th Annual Meeting; December 3-7.2004: New Orleans. Louisiana. Abstract 1.181.

19. Sheth RD, Drazkowski JF, Stanlo H et al. Unrecognised status epilepticus in the elderly. Program and abstracts of the American Epilepsy Society 58th Annual Meeting:December 3-7,2004;New Orleans Louisiana. Abstract 2.226.

20. Bromfield EB, Henderson GV. Treatment of seizures. *http://professionals. epilepsy.com/page/cerebrovas_treatment.html.* 1/02-.2010.

21. Ettinger AB. Diagnosing and treating epilepsy in the elderly. US Neurological Disease 2007. *http://www.touchneurology.com/diagnosing-treating-epilepsy-elderly-a7343-2.html* Accessed 11/14/2008.

22. Kwan P, Brodie MJ. Clinical trials of antiepileptic medications in newly diagnosed patients with epilepsy, *Neurology* 2003; 60 (suppl 4):S2-12 (abstract).

23. Reike S, Andreas S. Topiramate in elderly patients with epilepsy. Program and abstracts of the American Epilepsy Society 58th Annual Meeting December 3-7 2004, New Orleans, Lousiana. Abstract 2,358.

19

URINARY INCONTINENCE

AFTER STROKE

Introduction

Urinary incontinence (UI) is a common distressing and debilitating problem after stroke [1] and interferes with rehabilitation, delays recovery and discharge. UI in general has a negative impact on the quality of life [2,3] through multiple effects on daily activities or social functioning[4]. UI is associated medically with sepsis, recurrent urinary tract infections, decubitus ulcers[5], decreased mobility, dependency and depression. UI poststroke is a strong predictor of functional recovery[6]. Stroke survivors who are incontinent in the acute phase of the illness have a four-fold higher risk of institutionalization after a year [7].

Incidence prevalence and epidemiology

Several epidemiological studies have shown a high prevalence of urinary incontinence (UI) in the elderly patient especially women. It increases with age and was found to be 17% in men and 48% in women 70 years of age and women had 8 times higher odds of having UI than men when all ages 70-97 were pooled[8]. In poststroke patients in the acute phase the prevalence of UI is about 38.6% [9,10]. About 25% of the patients with post stroke UI still have problems on hospital discharge and 15%[11] to one-third remaining incontinent at one year[7]. The incidence of poststroke UI in patients over 75 years is higher than in patient's under 75 years[12] .

Pathophysiology

The corticoregulatory tract of micturition originates in the frontal cortex (areas 6 and 9) (controls bladder by contractions) and descends to the pontine micturition centre (coordinates detrusor contraction and uretheral relaxation) and to the Onuf's nuleus to finally synapse at the spinal cord centres in segments S2, S3 and S4 spinal segments at the lateral horn cells from where the pelvic nerves emanate. The bladder is innervated by sympathetic and parasympathetic nerves and are also controlled by higher cortical and subcortical centres, The sympathetic and parasympathetic have both afferent and efferent fibres.

According to Gelber et al[13] poststroke urinary incontinence is due to three major mechanisms. Firstly, disruption of the neuromicturition pathways resulting in bladder hyperreflexia and urge incontinence. The brain centres which control bladder contractions are compromised in stroke. This results in increased detrusor irritability, decrease cortical awareness of bladder filling and decrease voluntary control of the external sphincter[9].

Secondly, incontinence due to stroke-related cognition and language deficits with normal bladder function. Thirdly, concurrent neuropathy or medications causing underactive detrusor and overflow incontinence. Urodynamic studies are of benefit in establishing the cause of the incontinence. Gelber et al[13] reported the bladder to be hyper reflexic in 37% of 51 patients with recent unilateral ischaemic hemispheric stroke, 21% had bladder hyporeflexia and detrusor—sphincter dyssnergy. In another study most of the post stroke patients had overactive detrusor with or without detrusor sphincter dyssnergy[14.]

Studies have shown that the frontal lobe, basal ganglia and internal capsule lesions were associated with overactive bladder (OD) with or without detrusor—sphincter dyssnergy[15,16]. Based on neurophysiology OD without detrusor-sphincter dyssnergy is associated with suprapontine lesions and OD with detrusor—sphincter dysnnergy have suprasacral infrapontine lesions[14]. It has also been observed that stroke patients with lesions in the frontal lobe and basal ganglia had OD unihibited sphincter relaxation with the former and detrusor sphincter dyssnergy in the latter[16]. It is surmised that anteromedial frontal lobe and its descending pathway and the basal ganglia are mainly responsible for supranuclear type of pelvic and pudendal nerve dysfunction[16]. Neurological lesions between the brain stem (pontine micturition centre) and the sacral spinal cord are the cause of detrusor-external sphincter dyssnergia (sacral spinal centre[17]). The lesions are more usually caused by multiple sclerosis, transverse myelitis and traumatic spinal cord injury[17]. If detrusor sphincter dyssnergia is present in a stroke patient it is not likely to be due to an intracerebral lesion[6]. There is a strong correlation between UI and severity of the stroke with large infarcts, with aphasia and cognitive impaiment but not with age, sex, side of stroke or time of stroke[6].

Discussion

It is useful to categorise the problem into acute and chronic forms. The acute form is often remediable. The chronic forms are classified as urge, stress, mixed, overflow and functional. In UI stroke patients the fronto-parietal lobes and adjacent subcortical regions are likely to be affected. The sensory cortex including the attentional systems, cognition areas and emotional control areas are involved. Furthermore in the elderly in general frontal and global underperfusion and cognitive impairment are associated with urge incontinence together with reduced bladder sensation[18] .

Post-stroke UI has a significant negative impact on successful stroke rehabilitation and is a better indicator of negative functional outcome in haemorrhagic vs ischaemic stroke patients and patients with cortical vs subcortical lesions[12.] Several factors can influence continence and they include cognitive impairment, disordered sensorium, inability to communicate, decreased mobility among others[13,19] resulting in physical and psychological barriers to appropriate voiding. There is often impaired awareness which may range from slight unawareness to total denial of the leakage[20].

Assessment and Management

In most patients with the history, physical examination, urine analysis, urine culture and measurement of post-void residual urine (PVR) a diagnosis can be made (Fig 19.1). In a study of asymptomatic perimenopausal and postmenopausal women the investigators[21] found the PVR urine volume to be less than 50 ml in most of the women. According to the AHCPR Clinical guidelines for urinary incontinence in adults[22] a PVR of less than 50 ml is indicative of satisfactory bladder emptying and a PVR of more than 200ml unsatisfactory emptying. However there are no recommendation as to the implication of PVR between 50 ml and 200ml[22].

Treatment of poststroke UI includes behavioural and pharmacological interventions. In spite of the evidence for the different and effective interventions in treating urinary incontinence in the nonstroke elderly patients there is limited evidence in relation to stroke survivors[6]. If confusion can be reduced and mobility restored continence too will often return[23]. Patients who recognize their incontinence, attention focused training is an effective measure in re-establishing bladder control[24]. Behavioural techniques include Kegel's exercises, bladder training and bladder drill, prompted voiding, urge suppression and timed voiding. When they do not respond to behavioural techniques, anticholinergics and bladder training are options. Drugs with anticholinergic and smooth muscle relaxant properties (oxybutynin, solifenacin, imipramine, probantheline) are effective for urge incontinence. The side effects include dry mouth, constipation, and blurred vision. Imipramine can be used for both stress and urge incontinence. On the other hand cholinergics (bethanechol) and alpha-adrenergic blocker (prazosin) which stimulates bladder contractions and relax the sphincter are used in overflow UI. In those with overflow bladder life style changes such as reduction in weight and instruction in caffeine intake may help.

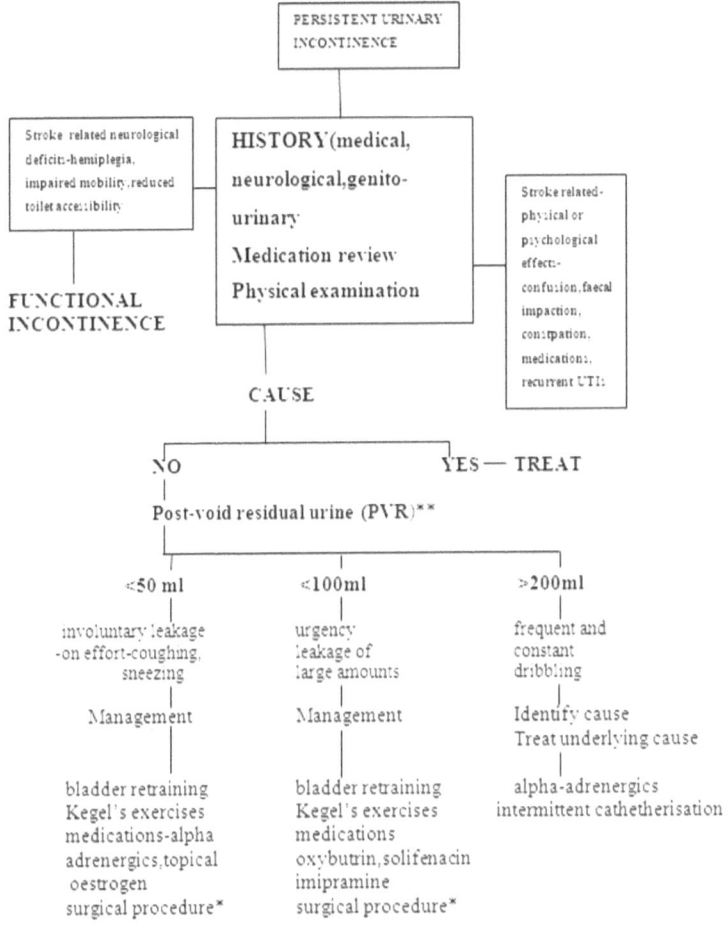

Fig. 19.1 Algorithm for evaluating poststroke urinary incontinence

* There a four-fold higher risk of institutionalization in stroke survivors who are incontinent in the acute phase of the stroke.
* Urinary incontinence has a strong correlation with stroke with large infarcts and aphasia and cognitive impairment but not with age, gender or sise of stroke.
* Post-stroke urinary incontinence has a negative impact on successful stroke rehabilitation.
* In most patients with the history, physical examination, urine analysis, urine culture and measurement of post-void residual urine (PVR) a diagnosis can be made.
* Measurement of the PVR urine volume should be part a full evaluation of a patient with UI.
* Treatment of poststroke UI includes behavioural and pharmacological interventions.
* In spite of the evidence for the different and effective interventions in treating urinary incontinence in the nonstroke elderly patients there is limited evidence in relation to stroke survivors.
* If confusion can be reduced and mobility restored continence too will often return[23]. Patients who recognize their incontinence, attention focused training is an effective measure in re-establishing bladder control.
* Behavioural techniques include Kegel's exercises, bladder training and bladder drill, prompted voiding, urge suppression and timed voiding.
* When they do not respond to behavioural techniques, anticholinergics and bladder training are options.

REFERENCES

1. Dumoulin C, Korner-Bitensky N, Tannenbaum C. Urinary incontinence in stroke. *Stroke* 2007;38:2745-2751.

2. Youn-Jong Son, Boeun Kwon. Predictive risk factors impaired quality of life in middle-aged women with urianary incontinence. *Int Neurourol J* 2010; 14(4):250-255 (abstract).

3. Chiaffarnio F, Parazzini F, LavezzaniM et al. Impact of urinary incontinence and overactive bladder on quality of life. *Eur Urol* 2003;43(5): 535-8 (abstract).

4. Leuderking WR, Nackley JF, Anderson RB, Testa MA. A review of the quality of life: aspects of urinary urge incontinence. *Pharmaeconomics* 1996;9(11):11-23.

5. Weiss BD. Diagnostic evaluation of urinary incontinence in geriatric patients *American Family Physician*,1998; 57(11):2675-2684.

6. Brittain KR, Peet SM, Castleden CM. Stroke and incontinence. *Stroke* 1998; 29: 524-8.

7. Kolominsky—Rabes PL, Hilz Max J, Neundoerfer B, Heuschmann PV. Impact of urinary incontinence after stroke. Results from a prospective population based stroke register. *Neurourology and Urodynamics* 2003; 22: 322-327.

8. Mollander U, Sundh V, Stein G. Urinary incontinence and related symptoms in older men and women studied longitudinally between 70 and 97 years of age. A population study. *Arch Geriatr Geront* 2002; 35: 237-244.

9. Reding MJ, Winter SW, Hochrein SA et al. Urinary incontinence after unilateral hemispheric stroke: A neurologic-epidemiologic perspective. *Neurorehab Neural Repair* 1987; 1: 25-30.

10. Brocklehurst JC, Andrews K, Richards B, Laycock PJ. Incidence and correlates of incontinence in stroke patients. *J Am Geriatr Soc* 1988; 33: 540-2

11. Thomas LH, Barrett J, Cross S et al. Prevention and treatment of urinary incontinence after stroke in adults. *Cochrane Database Syst Rev* (2005) (issue 3). Art no. CD004462. pub 2.

12. Turhan M, Atalay A, Atabak HK. Impact of stroke etiology lesion location and ageing on post-stroke urinary incontinence as a predictor of functional recovery. *Int J Reb Research* 2006; 29: 335-338.

13. Gelber DA, Good DC, Laven LJ, Verhulst SJ. Causes of urinary incontinence after acute hemispheric stroke. *Stroke* 1993; 24: 378-382.

14. Gupta A, Taly AB, Srivastava A, Thyloth M. Urodynamics post—stroke in patients with urinary incontinence: Is there correlation between bladder type and site of lesion? *Ann Indian Acad Neurol* 2009; 12: 104-7.

15. Kahn Z, Starer P, Yang WC, Bhola A. Analysis of voiding disorders in patients with cerebrovascular accidents. *Urology* 1990; 35: 205-70.

16. Sakakibara R, Hattori T, Yasuda K, Yamanishi T. Micturitional disturbance after acute hemispheric stroke. Analysis of the lesion site by CT and MRI. *J Neuro Sci* 1996: 137: 47-56(abstract).

17. Chancellor MB, Kaplan SA, Buivas JG. Detrusor-external sphincter dyssnergia. *Ciba Found Symp* 1990;151:195-206.

18. Griffiths DJ, McCraken PN, Harrison GM, Anne Gormley E, Moore KN. Urge incontinence and impaired detrusor contractility in the elderly. *Neurourol Urodyn* 2002.21:126-131.doi:10.1002/nau.10042.

19. Borrie MJ, Campbell AJ, Caradoc-Davies TH, Spears GF. Urinary incontinence after stroke: A prospective study. *Age Ageing* 1986; 15: 177-81.

20. Pettersen R, Haig Y, Nakstad PH, Wylller TB. Subtypes of urinary incontinence after stroke: relation to size and location of cerebrovascular damage. *Age Ageing* 2008; 37(3): 324-327.

21. Gehrich A, Stany MP, Fischer JRet al. Establishing a mean post void residual volume in asymptomatic perimenopausal and postmenopausal women. *Obstet Gynecol* 2007;110 (4):827-832.

22. United States Department of Health and Human Services agency for Health Care Policy and Research (AHCPR). Clinical practice guidelines. Urinary Incontinence in adults. Washington DC: United States department of Health and Humman Service Manual, 1992 as quoted by Gehrich et al [21].

23. Currie CT. Urinary incontinence after stroke. Brit Med J 1986: 293(6558): 1322-3.

24. Pettersen R, Saxby BK, Wylller TB. Poststroke urinary incontinence: one year outcome and relationship with measures of attentiveness. *J Am Geriatr Soc* 2007; 55(10): 1571-7.

20

Central post stroke pain

Introduction

In 1906 Dejerine and Roussy[1] described the thalamic pain syndrome which carried their name. Subsequently it was shown that the syndrome can occur with extrathalamic lesions. Foix et al[2] described cases due to cortical lesions and called it pseudo-thalamic syndrome. Others have described lesions elsewhere, in the bulbar[3], in the right parietal, and right mescenephalic regions[4]. For these reasons the term thalamic pain syndrome has been replaced by central post stroke pain (CPSP). It has since been shown that the term CPSP itself is unsatisfactory for it need not necessarily be due to a vascular lesion (infarct) and CPSP has been described with subarachnoid haemorrhage[5] and tumour[6].

Incidence prevalence epidemiology

Central post stroke pain (CPSP) affects between 2-6% of stroke patients that is, there is an annual incidence between 2000 and 6000 in the United Kingdom. Many of the patients with CPSP are younger than the general stroke population and may have it for several years giving a prevalence of 20,000 [5]. It is reported that approximately 30,000 survivors of stroke in the United States are affected by the so-called 'thalamic pain'[7]. Andersen et al[8] indicated an incidence of 6% among unselected stroke patients.

Pathophysiology

The neurophysiology of pain can be divided into four phases namely transduction, transmission, perception and modulation[9,10]. Transduction is the conversion of one form of energy to another be it chemical, thermal or mechanical into an electrochemical nerve impulse and made accessible to the brain. The afferent nocioceptors are at the free nerve endings of the primary nerve. The nociceptors have a cell body in the dorsal root ganglion and their axons are generally of two types, a thinly myelinated fibres (A-delta) and a smaller diameter non-myelinated (C-fibres).

The nociceptors have several different receptors on their surfaces and they include bradykinin, histamine, GABA and serotonin[11] which modulate the sensitivity of the stimulation. The axons synapse in the second order neurons in the dorsal horn of the spinal cord and some project through the ventral root[12].

Transmission is the way pain is transferred from peripheral to central nervous system. The major spinal pathway for pain crosses over to the anterolateral spinal quadrant to form the spinothalamic tract. The thalamic nuclei project to the somatosensory area of the cortex and the limbic and frontal lobes. The somatosensory cortex is involved in the localization and identification, and the limbic system and frontal lobe with the emotional aspects suffering or anxiety[13].

Perception is the awareness and both cortex and limbic system are involved in causing awareness of pain. The grey matter in the spinal cord is divided into ten laminae and the dorsal part constituting the laminae I to V deal with the in coming fibres. The modulating system is quite different from the sensory system and is differently organized, highly interconnected and appears to act as a unit[14]. This network and its pain suppressing action are organized at three levels of the neuraxis, the spinal cord, the medulla and mid brain[14]. Several supraspinal sites are involved in the descending control and including the midline periaqueductal gray-rostral ventromedial medulla (PAG-RVM) system[15]. The RVM particularly the nucleus raphe magnus modulates nociceptive transmission at the level of the dorsal horn of the spinal cord[16]. Pain signals pass through the dorsal horn via the ascending pathway to the periaqueductal gray and immediate adjacent midbrain.

Many of these signals never reach consciousness and are dampened by intrinsic modulatory activity. The gate control theory focuses on the descending pathway which has an important role in pain modulation[12] passes to the raphe nucleus in the upper medulla and then back to the dorsal horn via the reticulosopinal fibres and inhibit pain signaling.

Activation of the neurons in the midbrain periaqueductal gray matter excites neurons in the rostral medulla some of which contain serotonin. The medullary neurons in turn project to and specifically inhibit the firing of the trigeminal and spinal pain-tramission neurons[17]. Lesions at any level of the neuraxis generally involving the spinothalamic cortical afferent sensory pathways may produce pain including the cortex, subcortical white matter, thalamus, midbrain, pons and medulla[18,19,20].

The pathogenesis of CPSP remains unclear. It has been proposed that the spontaneous pain in CPSP is linked to hyperexcitability or spontaneous discharges in thalamic or cortical neurons that have lost their usual output[21]. CPSP has also been reported in association with lateral[22] and medial [23] medullary infarcts and it was postulated that the central pain is due to a selective 'neo' spinothalamic lesion' causing a 'denervation sensitivity of the 'paleo'-reticulothalamic connections[22].

Discussion

The pain in most instances develops within a week poststroke in 36% of patients. The frequency is 14% after thalamic lesions and 24% after geniculothalamic artery territory stroke[24]. The pain has been described as constant, intermittent, severe and burning and often tend to overact for noxious stimuli (hyperalgesia) and to non toxic stimuli (allodynia)[24]. The pain is confined to areas with sensory deficits[21] and there is a laterality predominance right over left.

Most patients with CPSP invariably show a deficit to pain and temperature sensations while touch and vibration are to a lesser extent affected. Somatosensory dysfunction was found in 42% of the population with stroke and pain is seen to occur only in patients with somatosensory dysfunction[8].

Wessel et al[25] in a study of 18 patients with ischaemic thalamic lesions correlated the clinical symptoms, somatosensensory evoked potentials (SEPs) and computed tomography (CT) findings. In most of their patients the thalamic lesions were either paramedian or anterolateral. According to them such differentiation is of prognostic value for those with loss of cortical SEPs and posterolateral ischaemic thalamic lesions on CT probably will not exhibit central pain.

Treatment

Browsher[5] recommends that the patients be treated initially with adrenergically active antidepressants (amitriptyline, nortriptyline, despramine, maprotiline) as soon as possible and emphasised that time should not be wasted trying conventional analgesics. If there is no response to antidepressants, mexitilene should be considered in suitable cases. Combined therapy with anticonvusants is acceptable and has been used[20]. Gabapentin has been found to be effective in neuropathic syndromes[26]. Pregabalin a structural congener of gabapentin causes problematic central nervous system adverse events such as somnolence and dizziness and hence is a concern in the elderly[27]. Lamotrigine is another anti-convulsant drug used in neuropathic pain. The side effects are dizziness, rash and sedation.

Balcofen an agonist of gamma-aminobutyric acid (GABA) receptor has antinociceptic effects. Balcofen injected intrathecally is said to give pain relief in patients with central pain due to stroke or spinal cord injury[28]. In one patient electrical stimulation of the pre-central gyrus gave satisfactory long lasting pain control (60-70% on visual analog scale)[4]. Implanted stimulators have a place in the patients resistant to medical treatment.

——————◆—————

* Central stroke pain affects between 2-6% of stroke patients.
* The pain in most instances develops within a week poststroke in 36% of patients.
* Occurs in thalamic and extrathalamic lesions.
* CPSP has also been reported in association with lateral and medial medullary infarcts.
* The pain is constant, intermittent, severe and burning and often tend to overact for noxious stimuli (hyperalgesia) and to non toxic stimuli (allodynia)[24].
* The pain is confined to areas with sensory deficits[21].
* Patients are treated with adrenergically active antidepressants initially and combined therapy with anticonvulsants is acceptable [5].

REFERENCES

1. Dejerine J, Rossy G. Le syndrome douloureux thalamique. *Rev Neurol (Paris)* 1906;14: 521-532.
2. Foix Ch, Chavany JA, Levy M. Syndrome pseudo-thalamique d'orgine parietale. Lesion de l'artere du silion interparieta. *CR Soc Neurol Paris* 1927; 168-75.
3. Ajuriaguerra J de. *La douleur dans les affections du systeme nerveux central.* Doin, Paris 1937.
4. Peyron R, Garcicia-Larrea L, Deiber MP. et al. Electrical stimulation of precentral cortical are in the treatment of central pain: electrophysiological and PET Study. *Pain* 1995; 62(3): 275-86.
5. Bowsher D. The management of central post-stroke pain. *Postgrad Med J* 1995; 71: 598-604.
6. Davison C, Schick W. Spontaneous pain and other sensory disturbances. *Arch Neurol Psychiat (Chicago)* 1935; 34: 1204-37.
7. Segatore M. Understanding central post-stroke pain. *J Neurosci Nurs* 1996; 28(1): 28-35.
8. Andersen G, Vestergaard K, Ingeman-Nielsen M, Jensen TS. Incidence of central post-stroke pain, *Pain* 1995; 61: 187-93.
9. Zacharoff LK. The Pathophysiology of pain. *http://www.nwrpca.org/health-center-news/156-the-pathophysiology-of-pain-ht retreived on 22.* 10.2012.
10. McCaffery M, Pasero C. Pain: A Clinical Manual. St Louis MO. Mosby,1990.
11. Wood S. Anatomy and physiology of pain. Nursing Times.net.Sept 26,2008.
12. Steed C.E. The anatomy and physiology of pain. *Surgery* 2009;27(12):507-511 (abstract).
13. Thamburaj AV. Physiology and management of pain. Global Spiner Network. *http://www.globalisoinal.net.physiology_of_pain* html. accessed on 11/16/2008.
14. Fields HL, Heinricher MM. Anatomy and physiology of nociceptive modulatory system. *Philos Trans R Soc.* Lond .B. Bio Sci.1985; 308: 361-374.
15. Heinricher MM, Tavares I, Leith JL, Lumb BM. Descending control of nociception: Specificity, recruitment and plasticity. *Brain Res Rev* 2009;60(1):214-225 (abstract).
16. Marinelli S, Viaghan CW, Schnell SA et al. Rostral ventromedial medulla neurons that project to the spinal cord express multiple opiod receptor phenotypes. *J Neurosci.* 2002; 22(24):10847-10855.
17. Basbaum AI, Fields H L. Endogenous pain control mechanisms: review and hypothesis. *Ann Neurol 1978* 1978;4(5):451-62 (abstract).
18. Beric A. Central pain: "new syndromes" and their evaluation. *Muscle Nerve* 1993; 16: 1017-1024.
19. Gonzales GR. Central pain. *Neurology* 1995; 45(suppl 9): 511-516.

20. Leigon G, Boivie J, Johanasson I. Central post-stroke pain: neurological symptoms and pain characteristics. *Pain* 1989; 36: 13-25.
21. Vestergaard K, Neilson J, Andersen G et al. Sensory abnormalities in consecutive unselected patients with central post-stroke pain. *Pain* 1995; 61: 177-186.
22. MacGowan DJ, Janal MN, Clark WC et al. Central poststroke pain and Wallenberg's lateral medullary infarction" frewuency, character and determinants in 63 patients. *Neurology* 1997;49(1):120-5.
23. Kim JS. Medial medullary infarct aggravates central poststroke pain caused by previous lateral medullary infarct. *Eur Neurol* 2007;58(1):41-3.
24. Nasreddine ZS, Saver JL. Pain after thalamic stroke: Right diencephalic predominance and clinical features in 1980 patients. *Neurology* 1997; 48: 1196-1199.
25. Wessel K, Vieregge P, Kessler C, Kompf D. Thalamic stroke: correlation of clinical symptoms, somatosensory evoked potentials and CT findings. *Acta Neurol Scand.* 1994; 90: 167-73.
26. Backonja M, Glanzman RL. Gabapentin dosing for neuropathic pain: evidence from randomized placebo-controlled clinical trials. *Clin Ther* 2003;25(1):81-104. (abstract).
27. Guay DR. Pregabalin in neuropathic pain: a more "pharmaceutically elegant" gabapentin. *Am J Geriatr Pharmacother* 2005;3(4):274-87. (abstract).
28. Taira T, Kawamura H, Tanikawa T et al. A new approach to control central deafferentation pain: spinal intrathecal baclofen. *Stereotact Funct Neurosurg* 1995; 65: 1201-5.

Index

Glossary of abbreviations

Chapter1
  IST-3—The third international stroke trial
  NINDS: National Institute of Neurological Disorders and Stroke
  SITS-MOST: The European Safe Implementation of Thrombolysis in Stroke
    Monitoring Study
  SITS-ISTR-International Stroke Thrombolysis Registry
  VISTA—Virtual International Stroke Trials Archive

Chapter 2
  ACA: anterior cerebral artery
  AICA: anterior inferior cerebellar artery
  CCA: common carotid artery
  ECA: external carotid artery
  GABA: gamma-aminobuytric acid
  ICA: internal carotid artery
  MCA: middle cerebral artery
  PCA: posterior cereral artery
  PICA: posterior inferior cerebellar artery

Chapter 3.
  ARIC study: Atheroscleosis Risk in Communities study
  AF: Atrial Fibrillation
  CHD: coronary artery disease
  CRP: C-Reactive Protein
  NEMESIS: North East Melbourne Stroke Incidence Study vWF: von
    Wiilibrand Factor

Chapter 4
  ADP: adenosine diphosphate
  CAA: Cerebral Amyloid Angiopathy

C BF: Cerebral Blood Flow
EAA: Excitatory aminacids
HI: Haemorrhagic Infarction
LDL: Low Density Lipoprotein
NMDA: N-methyl D-aspartate receptor
PH: Parenchymatous haematoma
PICH: Primary Intracerebral Haemorrhage
PCD:Programmed Cell Death

Chapter 5-7

AChA: Anterior chroidal artery
AICA: Anterior inferior cerebellar artery
DWMRI: Diffusion-Weighted Magnetic Reosonance Imaging
ICH: Intracerebral haemorrhage
PChA: Posterior chroidal artery
SCA: Superior cerebellar artery
SAH: Subarchnoid haemorrhage
TGA: Thalamic geniculate artery

Chapter 8

AIC: Acute isdchaemic stroke
DBP: Diastolic blood pressure
ECASS: European Co-operative Acute Stroke Study
IST-3: The third international stroke trial
Multi-MERCI study: Multi-Mechanical Emboli Removal in Cerebral Ischaemia
NINDS: National Instiute of Neurological Disordersa & Stroke
SEIS: Self expanding intractranial atherosclerotic stents
SITT-MOST study: European Safe Implementation of Thrombolysis in Stroke
    Monitoring Study BP: Systolic blood pressure tPA: tissue plasminogen
    activator rtPA: Recombinant tissue plasminogen activator rFVII:
    recombinant activated Factor VII

Chapter 9

CIMT: Constraint Induced movement therapy
FES: Functional electrical stimulation

Chapter 10

TIA: Transient ischaemic attack
TMB: Transient monocular blindness
EXPRESS study: Early Use of Existing Preventive Strategies for Stroke

Chapter 11-12

CA: carotid angiography

C-DUS: Carotid-Doppler Ultrasonography

CE-MRA: Contrast material Enhancer Magntic Resonance Angiography

CTA: Computed Tomographic Angiography

CEA: Carotid endarterectomy

CAS: Carotid artery stents

CREST: North Americam Carotid Revascularisation Endarterctomy Stenting Trial

ECST: European Carotid Surgery Trial

ESPS2: European Stroke Prevention Study2

MRA: Magnetic resonance angiography

TCD: Transcranial Doppler

Chapter 13

ACAS: Asymptomatic Carotid Atherosclerosis Surgery

ACST: Aysymptomatic Carotid Artery Stenting Trial

ACEI: Angiotensin Co-enzyme Inhibitor

CARDS: Collaborative Atovastin Diabetic Study

ETISH: European Trial on Isolated Systolic Hypertension in the Elderly

NASCET: North American Carotid Endarterectomy Trial

NVAF: Non-valvular atrial fibrillation

PVCs: Premarure ventricular complexes

PROGRESS:Perindopril Protective against Recurrent Stroke Study

SHEP study: Systolic Hypertension in the Elderly Progress study

Chapter 14-15

ACS: Acute confusional state

ACh: Acetyl choline

AM: Akinetic mutism

CBT: Cognitive behavioural therapy

GAD: Generalised anxiety disorder

ICAA: Inability to control anger

ICED: Involuntary emotional expression disorder

LOD: late onset depression

LOM: late onset mania

PDS: Poststroke depression

SSRIs: Selective serotonin receptor inhibitors

SCI: Silent cerebral infarction

TCAs: Tricyclic depressants

Chapter 16-20

AEDs: anti-epileptic drugs

CADASIL: Cerebral autosomal dominant arteriopathy with subcortical infarctions and leucoencephalopathies

CPSP: Central post stroke pain

FTD: Frontal lobe dementia

LADIS study: Leukoraiosis and Diability study VaD: Vascular Dementa

NCSE: non-convulsing status epilepticus

PLEDS: Periodic lateralizing epileptiform discharges

UI: Urinary incontinence

VCI: Vascular cognitive impairment

VaD: Vascular dementia

USEFUL ADDRESSES

AUSTRALIA
National Stroke Foundation
Head Office, Level 11,167 Queen Street
Melbourne, Victoria
Australia 3000
StrokeLine: 1800 786 653
Website: *www.strokefoundation.com.au*
Email: admin@strokefoundation.com.au

UNITED KINGDOM
Stroke Association
Stroke House
123-127Whitecross Street
London EC1Y 8J
UK
Tel: +44 (0) 20 7566 0300
Website: *http://www.stroke.org.uk*

UNITED STATES OF AMERICA
American Stroke Association
Website: http://www.strokeaha.org, http://www.strokeassociation.org